AF326574

"Andrew Barron's intimate and insightful reflections on life with his son Rafi, who has Down syndrome, challenges us to rethink disability and difference and what we ultimately value in life. In an age that often promotes detached speculation, sterilizes suffering, and worships efficiency, this storied approach to theological and ethical inquiry is a courageous invitation to elevate the importance of proximity and particularity and conceive of difference as normative, not abnormal."

—**PAUL LOUIS METZGER**, author of *More Than Things: A Personalist Ethics for a Throwaway Culture*

"Speaking powerfully out of his own experience with his son Rafi who lives with Down syndrome, Andrew Barron offers deep reflections on the sacredness of human difference and the hospitality of God. Readers won't agree with everything Barron says, but our disagreements are the beginning point for all vital transformative conversations. This book is an important contribution to the theology of disability."

—**JOHN SWINTON**, professor in practical theology and pastoral care, King's College, University of Aberdeen

"Thank God for Rafi Barron whose life has spurred his father to think deeply out of his combined Jewish and Christian set of commitments about the *difference that proximity* makes, and how being close to those who are different from us invites another posture of welcoming that much of conventional culture often otherizes. God's gifts through Rafi in these pages include probing reflections on the Bible and invitations to consider questions that we might not otherwise take up. Thanks be to God, and to Rafi!"

—**AMOS YONG**, author of *Theology and Down Syndrome: Reimagining Disability in Late Modernity*

"Andrew Barron's book engages directly with some of the most challenging and nagging issues of human life from and with God—family, suffering, death, incapacity, limitation, difference, divine love. It does so with compelling concreteness, at times gripping involvement, and always accessible prose, imagery, and argument. We won't agree with all the moves he makes, but we will ever be brought face to face with unavoidable divine questions, human imperatives, and acknowledged grace."

—**EPHRAIM RADNER**, professor emeritus of historical
theology, Wycliffe College, University of Toronto

"This book is much, much more than I expected on the subject of disability theology. This is a must-read for anyone who cares for someone who is disabled or different, who feels like an outsider because of their own difference, or who simply wants a fresh perspective on what it means to be a human person created in the image of God."

—**LORI BARON**, assistant professor of New
Testament, Saint Louis University

"Andrew Barron's book addresses the personal and spiritual challenges he and his family have encountered while journeying through life and faith with Rafi, who has Down syndrome. With a combination of honesty, integrity, and faith, Barron delves into profound and heart-searching questions using insights from Jewish and Christian thought, theology, and contemporary studies on difference and disability."

—**RICHARD HARVEY**, associate lecturer, All Nations Christian College

Human Difference

Human Difference

Reflections on a Life in Proximity to Disability

Andrew Barron

Foreword by Ephraim Radner

CASCADE *Books* · Eugene, Oregon

HUMAN DIFFERENCE
Reflections on a Life in Proximity to Disability

Cascade Books
An Imprint of Wipf and Stock Publishers
199 W. 8th Ave., Suite 3
Eugene, OR 97401

www.wipfandstock.com

PAPERBACK ISBN: 978-1-6667-7923-3
HARDCOVER ISBN: 978-1-6667-7924-0
EBOOK ISBN: 978-1-6667-7925-7

Cataloguing-in-Publication data:

Names: Barron, Andrew, author. | Radner, Ephraim, foreword.

Title: Human difference : reflections on a life in proximity to disability / Andrew Barron.

Description: Eugene, OR: Cascade Books, 2024 | Includes bibliographical references.

Identifiers: ISBN 978-1-6667-7923-3 (paperback) | ISBN 978-1-6667-7924-0 (hardcover) | ISBN 978-1-6667-7925-7 (ebook)

Subjects: LCSH: People with disabilities—Religious aspects—Christianity. | Human body—Religious aspects—Christianity. | Church work with people with disabilities.

Classification: BV4460 B40 2024 (paperback) | BV4460 (ebook)

VERSION NUMBER 08/02/24

This is for Laura, Rafi, Ketzia, and Simona. Your devotion and confidence and love are the most valuable things I have.

Contents

Foreword

THIS BOOK IS ABOUT divine blessing and the joyful, if sometimes perturbing, fruit of such blessing's recognition. Cast as a reflection on divine creation emerging from his life with his son Rafi, born with Down syndrome, Barron invites us to "consider the works" of God's "hands" with a grateful wonder that reaches down into the realities of each of our own times and places, encounters, and relations.

Barron begins his first chapter, "Reflections on a Life in Proximity," with an epigraph from Maimonides, based on the Talmud. It is the blessing of God one is to give upon seeing something unusual, in this case an unusual human being: "Blessed are You, Lord our God, King of the universe, who makes people different." One might say this blessing on first encountering someone from a foreign race, or of a strange build or figure. Yet, the encounter is to draw forth praise and wonder before the Lord of heaven and earth.

Barron's larger vision flows from this fundamental command: our life's meaning is comprehensively wrapped up with receiving this life, with all its encounters, as a gift from God. This life, in its proximities to every sort of thing or person, is the revelation of God as love. The metaphysics implied here are vast: "what is" is what we receive from God. And hence the purpose of our life is to apprehend this and live in and as this gift's acknowledgment. Reception and thanksgiving undergird the whole of our existence as persons with other persons, something Barron alludes to in his discussion of the Eucharist as participation even in the broken body of Jesus.

The talmudic blessing upon which Barron hangs his narrative comes from a set of blessings under the heading of *meshane habriyot*, exclamations of thanks to the God who "creates difference," or perhaps more literally, who "changes [i.e. alters] creatures." The wonder here is the divine act and will in creation itself, at the beginning of all things, as in Genesis, but also at every point in the life of the world and its inhabitants. In the rabbinic tradition, this blessing forms part of the series of blessings on "sightings," on seeing new and unusual things—elephants, monkeys, and, as mentioned, different forms of human life in terms of race or body—things that *God* has made, yet that are marvelous, if beyond our sense of order.

This kind of response to what lies around us, including people, delights in receiving the world as a gift. But it is an attitude that is deeply antithetical to a more general modern sense of life as a projection of myself onto what is "out there." Most of us live in a way that yearns and works for the conformity of the world to our own desires—good desires, one hopes, but ours, nonetheless. Our world tends, in our imaginations, to be a place of becoming according to our hopes, principles, and standards. Hence, our projection of God's truth and gift ever into the future—what heaven must be like, how the nations of the world must be reformed. Even the modern press for "improving" the lives of others—politically, ethically, in appearance even—springs out of this self-originated impulse. But in this, the reality of life itself—its givenness by God and its thankful reception—is obscured. Much of what God offers us, we run from.

Barron's wonderfully illuminating account steadfastly breaks away from this trend. With his son Rafi as its dynamic center, the wonderful givenness of life, in all its particularities and "differences," is exposed as a divine gift. Rafi has his struggles, and so does his family, and Barron has also in his own way as Rafi's father. But Rafi is a single person, not a "type"; he has his own personality, his own experiences, his own feelings, and ways of thinking, sometimes difficult for others to penetrate or understand, but "all his." The energies of this volume derive from this singular story, and it would be worth telling on its own. In fact, just *this* story on its own is partly what Barron wants to help us see as profoundly valuable.

But Barron tells us a parallel story, the story of his own reordering of vision by the grace of seeing and by the press of human nearness—"proximity," as he likes to tell us; nearness to the wondrous if disorienting creative work of God in others who are not "like us" in so many ways. To watch closely and live closely with Rafi—a father with his son, but just *this* son—is to be opened up to God, and to a world that God has made that is quite different from the self-projecting norms of much of our artificially steadied lives.

Barron's book engages directly with some of the most challenging and nagging issues of human life and of that life as a life from and with God—family, suffering, death, incapacity, limitation, frustration, unexpected joy, difference, divine love. It does so with compelling concreteness, at times gripping involvement, and always accessible prose, imagery, and argument. Finally, Barron takes on these realities of life in a way that is saturated in a biblical openness and faith. And all this from the perspective of God's creating marvels. "Difference"—Rafi as "different," but also a crowd of others whom Barron meets and comes to know—becomes a "blessed" cracking open of the world—our self-made or self-satisfied or simply self-exhausted worlds of habit—to God's work, and thus God's life. Once opened up in this way, the world doesn't just "look different" than it appears in our sullen self-enclosures; it is *filled* with infinite marvels that reorder our sensibilities not simply as a means of play, but as a landscape of understanding and experience. Barron's discussion, for instance, of Rafi's sense of "time" is a revelation of existential truth that is both haunting and liberating.

There is a fragile balance that Barron needs to navigate in this act of gentle, but engrossing narrative. How to maintain the astonishing recognition of the divine gift of particularity that is Rafi's, while also commending the recognition as a practice, one that others can identify and assume in a regular and hence repeatable way? The temptation to turn singularities into conceptually undifferentiating categories—disability, the marginalized, and so on—is hard to avoid, even as they necessarily reduce precisely what makes "difference" always a divine *sui generis* of wonder and grateful exclamation.

On the whole, Barron is successful here. But I would myself demur, for example, from his argument on same-sex blessing and marriage as an acknowledgment and respect for "difference." The logic seems to be that what is "good" for a heterosexual person—marriage in this case—should morally be extended to everyone, no matter their "difference." But that makes difference a kind of demand for sameness, and places us back on the unending conveyor belt that would remake the world into its future uniformities. Once "difference" becomes a principle to be applied to social life, it inevitably takes on the force of imposed uniformity.

The Jewish blessings of difference are in fact distinguished between the changes or diversities that God has made and those that we make of ourselves and others. Social and moral "norms," as Barron rightly notes, are not principles in this way. At their best, they are both practical means by which it is possible for most people to learn how to live with one another, gain the skills of recognition, and forego the coercive drift of self-manufacture imposed on others. Rightly applied, moral norms sketch the boundaries within which difference—God's work—can be recognized and respected broadly, if not, alas, always precisely.

Of course, this last aspect is where Barron's larger argument remains so important: our application of norms has not always permitted such respectful recognition, and in fact in many cases has squelched it. The center of the divine work of difference-making is the self-giving of God in his Son, as the Messiah who takes flesh, who "comes close" to us in the most intimate proximity that the Lord of all things might offer, in the womb of a human mother, and born into the world of men and women. He is given a name, and lives in just this family, not another, not every family. He eats and works and interacts in the specific moments and details that no one else can share, and that are in fact obscure to us today.

Yet this creating God thereby lives a "normal" life that, at the same time, breaks open the realm of expectation with teaching, healing, astonishing honesty, and forgiveness, and finally with his own humanly unacceptable suffering and death. In doing this, the world's contours, in their variegated particularity, are thrown upon to "view," to "sighting," to the light: lepers, prostitutes, the lame, the possessed and mentally burdened, even the dead and the smell of their rotting flesh. That this Messiah should then rise from such a place of numbed sameness, to be touched just in his wounded flesh, in just this or that place of the nails and gashes, is to infuse the Lord's "diverse creation" with his own particular self, upon whose back, as it were, the whole universe can now be viewed with eyes of thanks rather than resentful self-protection and promotion.

Barron's book is a deeply Christian volume, exploring who God is, and who God is in particular in Jesus of Nazareth, the Messiah. The particularities of Rafi's life end up forming a singular echo of divine life. Human history, rightly viewed as Barron does, is always a form of theology proper.

Human Difference is ultimately the story of faith. Barron's own coming to faith was itself an instance of this intimate divine proximity—this apotheosis of difference—as he, a somewhat aimless Jew "came to believe in God and that Jesus was the Messiah of the Jewish people and the Savior" while remaining, somehow, still "Jewish." A wonder in its own right, a "sight" for which God's work of change is to be blessed: "For my father is always at his work to this very day, and I too am working" (John 5:17 [NIV]). Because of this, the story of Rafi, of Andrew Barron and his family, of the world in which they live, is one of tremendous joy. This volume proves that testimony, at its most honest, most reflective, most open is not just a personal witness, but an actual revelation of the Spirit to the God, not only of "unsearchable judgments" beneath which we cower, but of unbounded "riches of wisdom" in which we are called to delight (Rom 11:33). Blessed by God who makes a world of diverse creatures.

Dr. Ephraim Radner
Professor of Historical Theology
Wycliffe College University of Toronto

Acknowledgments

This book wouldn't have seen the light of day if it were not for Ephraim Radner, Michael Thomson, and Faydra Shapiro. Thank you.

Disclaimer

This book is a work of nonfiction. While the events described herein are based on actual occurrences, certain names, identifying details, and circumstances have been altered to protect the privacy and confidentiality of the individuals involved. Any resemblance to persons, living or deceased, or actual events, beyond those disclosed, is entirely coincidental.

This disclaimer is provided to clarify that while the core narrative remains true to real-life events, the protective measures taken may result in some minor deviations from actual events or characters. The primary objective is to honor the trust placed in the author by the individuals whose experiences have been recounted.

Introduction

A 2 AM PHONE call from the hospital is rarely good: "I think you should get down here right away." Rafi had been born a few hours earlier, and I had gone home to get a little rest, although only after calling family and friends to share our exciting news.

When I insisted on knowing why, the doctor explained—hesitatingly—that he thought our newborn son might have Down syndrome.

I promptly jumped into the shower and vomited.

Whose life was this?

Shaking violently, I was acutely aware that if it turned out that I couldn't handle this news, then everything I thought about myself to be true, was in fact a lie. Entering the hospital, I felt keenly that I was crossing a threshold, that my life was about to be changed forever. I stood on the doorstep of difference. The pediatrician and I shook hands, and together we walked in to meet with my wife.

Laura and I had been living in South Africa for six years, where we had moved just a few months after our wedding. We worked long hours and enjoyed everything that the country could offer. It was a remarkable life: we made many friends, traveled to exotic places. We lived there through a historic moment: Nelson Mandela had been released from prison shortly after we arrived. It was exciting and charming. It was shocking and sad. It was beautiful and ugly. The contradictions were in our face every day. The relationships were intense, and we loved it all. We thought about staying long-term.

Then Rafael came into our lives.

It's funny how much difference an extra chromosome makes.

Laura's pregnancy had been normal. We had no reason to expect that Rafi would be the kind of different that would so profoundly affect the trajectory of his life. And ours. His particular difference lay in his chromosomal composition; those small bundles of genes have a lot to say about how the body and mind develop. All those differences were already present when he was conceived and lay curled within, invisible to us. There Rafi was, inside my wife, already who he is. There had been no reason for extensive medical tests: Laura was young and healthy. All the indicators were normal.

I often wonder what those months would have been like if we knew of the difference that lay quietly waiting to emerge.

Twenty-six years later, Rafi's difference is clearly present in his orientation to his own body, to time, to space. I am not sure if he really knows what time it is or where he is. He is not good with abstractions. He can read the time, and he is always in the present. He knows he lives in Toronto and he looks at maps, but I am not sure he knows where he is. His body, too, seems a mystery. It's soft and mushy and he has very little muscle tone. He is comfortable being naked around strangers and helpers. He is not ashamed to burp, fart, slurp, or laugh around anyone at any time. He smiles easily, but he is not always in a good mood. He complains if things are out of order. Once we were in a bookstore together when Rafi bumped into an extremely tall man. He looked up and with astonishment said "Wow!" The man smiled and the two of them enjoyed a good laugh together, an affectionate moment of sympathy in mutual differences.

Rafi seems impervious to sorrow. Friends, family, and animals we know and loved, have died over the years without much reaction. He calls his new dog the same name as his old dog. He speaks of dead relatives in the present tense. Where are grandpa and grandma? In Florida! And where is that? Florida is right next door to Rafi. Everything is present, in space and in time.

This lack of orientation acutely affects his life and ours and definitively establishes difference in our lives from those of our friends and peers. Rafi can never be alone. He cannot respond to an emergency. He cannot organize his day, toilet himself, or walk alone to the park. He has echolalia: He repeats the last thing you say. Did you go to the park? Yes. Did you go to the store? Yes. One or either (or neither) might be true. The day he underwent dental surgery, we ate dinner together that evening. What did you do today, Rafi? I went to Walmart. He is loving, funny, adorable, charming, infuriating.

We always need to know where he is and what he is doing. He understands that money is necessary, but only in an abstract way. He cannot make life decisions. His receptive language is excellent. His descriptive language is minimal. He doesn't have friends in the same way the rest of us do. All the people he regularly spends time with—outside of family—are paid. He loves to talk, but mostly about the next meal to come or what the previous one was.

Rafi's memory is astounding. He recalls restaurants and meals in a way like my father did. My father had this unusual ability: We would be driving and pass a restaurant when my father would say something like "I had a really good pastrami sandwich there back in 1968, but they didn't toast the rye bread enough and the mustard was too tangy." How many meals do you need to remember? For Rafi and my father, quite a few.

The hospital in Johannesburg where he had been born was terrific and Rafi underwent a whirlwind of tests. We were filled with nervous anxiety as his heart was checked, but it seemed a normal day all around us as the doctor casually gossiped with the nurses. Everything passed in slow motion. He is fine, don't worry. Of course you're stunned. Take him home and take care of him. He is going to do well. He will surprise you. He looks like you.

We received awkward calls from friends all over the world: *Congratulations . . . I'm so sorry.* As we waited to make sure he was okay, we were asked about circumcision. It was the last thing on my mind, but I'm glad someone thought of it. A kind urologist from Scotland with training in this ancient Jewish rite took Rafi away and came back later to show off his handiwork. "If you have any questions about his penis, please call me," he said, handing me his card. I laughed for the first time since Rafi's birth.

When we were finally released home, it was a struggle for Rafi to latch on to breastfeed. His muscle tone was just too weak. We had to feed him through a tube in his nose, but when the food hit his stomach his eyes lit up, just the same way they do today. With the help of a great nurse whose stubbornness matched Rafi's own, he slowly figured out the connection between his mouth and his belly. We laughed and cried when he finally latched on and ate with abandon. After that he grew quickly, but he was undoubtedly delayed.

No one really treated Rafi differently. He was carried here and there, he played, he laughed, he thrived. Sure, his milestones were different from those of other kids, but what did it matter? He was Rafi. Things would take as long as they took. He was different and he was ours. We embraced it all. Our aging parents were in the United States, and we were too far from them in South Africa. So we moved to Canada, anticipating better disability resources there.

After Rafi was born we had two girls, and they grew up thinking his difference was normal. "What? Not everyone has a brother with Down syndrome?" Rafi went to school and was popular, but he didn't have any real friends. No one tried to include him in the street hockey or basketball being played in the neighborhood.

Rafi is now an adult. He attends a vocational day program and works at a pet store and a restaurant, leaving early in the morning and returning home in the late afternoon. His helpers come on weekends to swim, play basketball and tennis. Some help him shower and shave. He is a man, and it is hard to know how to manage a man who sometimes acts like a toddler.

We have been through a lot of behavioral problems. Rafael can be angry, belligerent, petulant. He can become compulsive about his eating and daily schedule. He sometimes refuses to get on or off his bus. He might freeze up or shut down. He once punched his helper. We spent thousands of dollars on therapists, but when we asked Rafi about what was going on he would answer "I don't know." He understood that we were concerned, but he could not communicate what was going on internally. The best the doctors could do was diagnose depression and anxiety based on his symptoms.

I could list the things that Rafi is missing out on: independence, intimacy, travel, money, vocation. But he is not really missing out on anything. He is loved and he loves. He has a sense of belonging. He is cared for. I do not think I want Rafi to have Down syndrome. Yet days and weeks go by where I don't even think about it. Our lives have a pattern much like everybody else's. If Rafi were "normally" developed, our lives would simply be different, not better. Our own contentedness flowers from being securely planted inside this space of difference.

Workbook Questions

1. The author remembers that he "felt keenly that I was crossing a threshold, that my life was about to be changed forever." Have you had a moment like this in your own life, where you realized that everything you think to be true about yourself is about to be put to the test?

2. How do you think things would have been different had Andrew and Laura known in advance that they would be having a child with Down syndrome? Would that have been easier or more difficult?

3. Putting yourself in the role of friend to Andrew and Laura—what would you have liked to say to them on hearing about the birth of Rafi?

4. "I could list the things that Rafi is missing out on." Can we imagine what the disabled might see the able-bodied as missing out on?

1

Reflections on a Life in Proximity

One who sees . . . people with disfigured faces or limbs, recites the
blessing, "Blessed are You, Lord our God, King of the universe, who
makes people different." One who sees a person who is blind or
lame . . . recites the blessing, "Blessed are You, Lord our God, King of
the universe, who is a righteous judge." But if they were born that way
[with the disability], one says, "who makes people different."

—Maimonides, Mishneh Torah, Laws of Blessings, 10:12

I WAS ELEVEN WHEN I interviewed my grandmother for a project in grade
school. I did not know her very well, and this was a chance to learn something about her immigrant experience. What made her get on a boat at the
age of fourteen and emigrate from Poland to the United States? Her answer
was simple: "Because we were different." But I never thought of myself as
particularly different. The Jewish neighborhood of Bayside, Queens in New
York City was full of people like me: second- or third-generation American
Jews living in multigenerational houses.

I was an average kid, going about the business of growing up with
others who were mostly like me.

It was many years later that an encounter startled me into thinking
seriously about difference.

I was at a family wedding, eagerly scanning for someone to talk to so I wouldn't have to mingle, when a woman approached me with a warm-hearted and welcoming smile. Her face was familiar, and she introduced herself with me a handshake that I remember to this day: eyes straight, warm, firm, and affectionate.

"Do you remember me? You knew me as . . . Paul." It was like seeing someone from a distance and only slowly as they walk toward you do their features properly sharpen into focus. "Yes!" But then I found myself awkward and unsure of what to say next. It was her own familiarity with these conversations that rescued me. "It's okay. My name is Kristen. I'm not the person you remember." She was so kind and patient with me I could have wept in shame.

Kristen reminded me that we attended Hebrew school together and had celebrated our bar mitzvahs the same year. As she spoke, I recuperated, got my bearings, and found myself liking her enormously. She was immediate, funny, honest, and transparent. She specifically wanted to speak to me, it turned out, because she had heard that I "believe in God" and had "become religious." So, we sat together.

Kristen told me that it was just after bar mitzvah that he told his siblings that he was a woman. They insisted he not tell their parents: they were traditionally minded and he was afraid of shaming them. So here's what Paul did: he got a secure job after high school and kept expenses down in order to save all he could. He kept to himself and waited. Twenty years or so later, when his parents were both gone, he was ready. He was quiet, modest, and deliberate. He took the time he needed: research, doctors, therapy, applications, humiliation. He went through surgery (top and bottom) and grueling pain, physiotherapy, and counseling. He went through this long and painful process and here she was at the other end of it. Kristen was happy, secure, in a relationship, and spiritually hungry. I was in awe and bewildered.

"Can I ask you some personal questions?" She was open and ferociously transparent. (What exactly did they do to your body? Did it hurt? How does your body work now? How does it feel? How does the plumbing work? Who are you on the inside, sex and with whom, and what about masturbation?) Her openness took my breath away. She wanted to show me, but I demurred. She answered without hesitation or embarrassment. Her story was at once heartbreaking and redemptive. Physical pain that at the time was almost unbearable had become a memory of endurance, commitment, and perseverance. She was not going to give up. She said that she just wanted to be herself. Is she disordered or is she different? The commonness of our humanity was the place of recognition that we were not so different. Being in proximity to difference changes you.

It is important to state that I do not honor the difference I have with my friend in a way that evaporates into a kind of mushy relativism. There is another side, one that I can keep in tension: I believe that we all must be oriented and ordered toward the God of Israel and his Messiah Jesus. I assert that the God of Israel is the living God and, ipso facto, all other gods are idols. But within our individual lives, God superintends, is active and guides us alongside and inside diversity. So, while no person is identical to another, we do not celebrate all human expressions simply because of difference. Rather difference is celebrated insofar as it is oriented to God. Jesus inhabits all that difference.

What does that mean for my friend Kristen and for Rafi, and where is the line to be drawn? Where do descriptions end, and proscriptions begin? My time spent in proximity to the difference has taught me to give more and more generous space: a wider berth. God judges justly. Kristen needs the God of Israel and so does Rafi and so do I. Kristen is broken sexually and so am I. Rafi, well, I do not know. I do not think Rafi knows what sex is. He talks about his penis, and he knows I have one. He knows that his mother and sisters don't, but sexual organs are neutral to him. "Does God care what I do with my penis?" is not something that Rafi wonders about. I am skeptical of absolutes regarding difference. I know that some will disagree. I can only wish for those who disagree to spend as much time with difference as I do.

At the wedding, Kristen asked to hear my story: how I came to believe in God and that Jesus was the Messiah of the Jewish people and the Savior. How was I still Jewish? We noticed that our stories were similar in a way—both provocative and controversial, at once paradoxical and dissonant. And joyful. Something significant happened and we both changed on the inside and outside. "What I really want to know is how to believe in God." She asked me to pray for her and I did so, in the middle of a wedding reception, praying that she would know God and that he would comfort her and reveal himself to her. It was clear to me that my friend and I were not so different.

Difference

I would like you to read this book, but if you get no further than this, here is what I want you to remember: closeness to people who are different from you—in disability, in worldview, in faith, in any of the myriad ways that humans are different—teaches you things you could not learn otherwise.

It is easy to live in echo chambers of our own making, where we have sought out people with whom we have much in common and with whom we agree. Social media exacerbates this tendency to cluster with people whose similar religious faith, political leanings, age, or stage allow us to feel supported. Yet there are obvious downsides to these cocoons of similarity. In this kind of environment, we need to be particularly intentional in seeking out difference.

Being in proximity to difference transforms our mental categories: how we see and think about the world and how we think, how we ask questions and how you reflect on stories. When Jean Vanier went to live in community of the physically and intellectually different, he said that "it has been this life together that has helped me become more human."[1]

This happened to me, and I am thankful.

This is a book about human difference and disability. I have come to believe more and more that we live in a world of human difference, and we must seek to understand that and embrace the uncertainty that comes with it. I want to reflect on how we might better cope with and ultimately be enriched by its ambiguity. I have written this manifesto for myself, in order to be more fully human.

A word on terminology. We often use "disability" as a collective representation for difference. It is an implied social contract that implies that certain things are normal and certain things are not. This category is indeed useful for some people to gain access to services and have their needs met. But disability is only one aspect of human difference. In discussing these artificial constructs, John Swinton notes that "when we make these things up that very often, they become quite negative, quite pathological.

---

1. Vanier, *Becoming Human*, 6. In February 2023, a nine-hundred-page independent report commissioned by L'Arche concluded that Vanier sexually abused at least twenty-five adult women between 1950 and his death in 2019. I have been and continue to be nourished and inspired through Vanier's writing and his example of a life dedicated to the disabled. In Jewish tradition we say these things when a person dies: *may his memory be for blessing . . . blessed be the true Judge*. It is up to us to remember it all. Vanier's legacy, although tarnished, continues in the good work of this organization that is dedicated to the disabled and different. That memory is a blessing for good.

So, disability for me is a way of naming difference, but not necessarily the best way of naming difference."[2] Sometimes I will use terms "disability" and "difference" interchangeably.

I would never imply that all aspects of human difference are forms of human disability. Nor would I accept that human difference which harms others can be justified. By "difference" I mean those states or attributes that interpersonally or socially divide and separate groups of persons from other persons. In many cases, the body reveals such difference, albeit in varying degrees and forms. While in American society eye color has little differentiating power, skin color has enormous differentiating power.[3] The way we receive physical characteristics is both deeply unequal and culturally encoded in society,[4] although in different ways across times and places, all human societies understand bodies as indicators of difference. Difference can be offensive.

How Does It Feel to Be a Problem?

W. E. B. DuBois asked this question in *The Souls of Black Folk*, writing about the alienation experienced by African Americans. He described the isolation and distance he felt: "It dawned upon me with a certain suddenness that I was different from the others; or like, mayhap, in heart and life and longing, but shut out from their world by a vast veil."[5]

Rafi and I were at a dance night for people with special needs. I was sitting on a bench outside the dance floor next to a woman and her helper. When the helper got up to get a drink the woman took my hand and began signing on it. She was blind and deaf, but she sought out connection. She was talking to me, and I could not understand her. Later, when her helper returned, they talked. I was the outsider—it was I who was different. I who was shut out.

2. Swinton, "Breaking the Mold."

3. This recognition is compounded when the context is changed to National Socialist Germany. Clearly there, eye color had far more differentiating power.

4. One might also note a similar contrast in social reception of physical augmentation/enhancement. For example, some would interpret the act of receiving dental implants for degenerating teeth quite differently from breast augmentation. In this case, dental implants are far less likely to be perceived as "vain" or reflective of some negative personality characteristic.

5. Du Bois, "Strivings," 194.

History bursts with disastrous examples of how to manage the "problem of difference." The ancient world knew about human difference and tried to come to terms with it. I think they were mostly afraid of it. We don't have much access to information about social attitudes in the ancient world, so we cannot understand a lot about their approaches to the disabled. We can say however that they saw disability difference as a bad omen—there was a supernatural quality to difference: difference and disability was tied into the judgments of the gods. People who were different were weak.

Human difference, particularly when it presents in the body, is felt to demand a story, an explanation, on the part of those with "normal" bodies:

> Just as disability is a difference with a difference (and in some ways more fundamental than differences in race, ethnicity, and genre), it stands in a unique relation to life narrative . . . [D]eviations from bodily norms often provoke a demand for explanatory narrative in everyday life. Whereas the unmarked case—the "normal" body—can pass without narration, the marked case—the scar, the limp, the missing limb or the obvious prosthesis—calls for a story. People presenting unexpectedly anomalous bodies are often called upon to account for them, sometimes explicitly: "What happened to you?" . . . One of the social burdens of disability, then, is that it exposes affected individuals to inspection, interrogation, and violation of privacy.[6]

But inside of us all there is no normal. There are predispositions, tendencies, and biases. The norm in fact is difference, and we choose what kinds of difference are acceptable. There are many ways to be normal and our ideas of it shape our personal and cultural thinking. "Difference" is not a neutral term—it is deeply theological and social and anthropological. It goes to the heart of what it means to human.

What is difference? When we think of human difference we tend to focus on the disabled. When it comes to human difference the disabled different are "perhaps the most fundamental; and in many places the least recognized, the least remembered, and the most life threatening"[7] group of people with a named difference. But disability is only one piece of the puzzle of difference. Swinton asserts that

> disability is simply a cultural marker for difference. It is a consensus that we come to that certain thing are normal and certain things

6. Couser, "Disability as Diversity," 105.

7. Couser, "Disability as Diversity," 111.

are not normal . . . If you had a society that was not particularly interested in intellect, it was more interested in community . . . then the category "intellectual disability" would be meaningless. So, although it is necessary perhaps for to access certain services and to help people to have their meet the needs met, it's just something that people make up. And it's when we make these things up that very often, they become quite negative . . . So, disability for me is a way of naming difference, but not necessarily the best way of naming difference.[8]

Swinton's challenge is clear to me: Human difference is a construction based on a society's priorities and interests. Yet I freely acknowledge that we often benefit from these very constructions, from the category "disabled" to take care of Rafi. Access to money, resources, and technology have been a blessing to us and have added to the quality of his life. When Rafi was a child, we received "parent relief" income. When Rafi became an adult, he qualified for disability income. We submitted his doctor's testimony and filled out an application that had a lot of boxes. The more boxes we checked, the more money we received. That is the way it works. Those classifications might be made up, but they also matter.

For those with differences that constrain, there are real needs to be addressed. The person receiving the benefit, however, is reduced to a "client" or a "patient," which can easily become a kind of diminishment. (After all, a "patient" is one who endures, who is long-suffering.) You're in a hospital for a procedure or test? You are asked to change into a gown, and you reenter the world lessened. You are exposed. You become a passive object and a recipient. A client needs something and is in a position of subordination in relation to the person or institution that has authority to dispense it. The client is diminished. The charitable model sees disability as victimhood, a difference that is "tolerated." Surely it is a good to use community resources to help and protect and defend. But after a person is helped and protected and defended, then what do they do? How are they included? How do they belong?

The model of "tolerance" towards difference is in fact often quite intolerant because "the tolerant" want to control and have the different behave according to standards established by the tolerant. In a 1790 letter to the Jewish community of Newport, Rhode Island, George Washington wrote: "It is now no more that toleration is spoken of, as if it was by the

---

8. Swinton, "Breaking the Mold."

indulgence of one class of people that another enjoyed the exercise of their inherent natural rights."[9] Washington knew that people are different and that too often the normal are given the power and make decisions about the abnormal.

The Problem of Difference

We were in an ER one day and the doctor said, "Besides Down syndrome what else is the problem?" I said that Rafi has a urinary infection. And that Down syndrome is not a problem. I could tell he was embarrassed and reflective. I would like to think his outlook was shaken up a little. Down syndrome is not something that is broken or wrong or needs to be fixed. It does not define Rafi. He is a human being trying to get by with the help of his family and friends, like most of us.

Being independent, "standing on your own two feet," not being a burden—these are considered markers of adulthood in our modern Western society. I remember teaching Mary, Rafi's new helper, how to go through Rafi's bathroom routine. He needs help showering, shaving, toileting. Rafi is a grown man: use your imagination. Her eyes got big. But for him it is normal and natural to be taken care of this way. I told her that she should not have any embarrassment: "Your job is to assist him. His job is to be assisted." Most of us toilet, shave, shower, and get dressed without help, routines that take as long as they take. Rafi follows his routines with help. They take as long as they take.

We insist that managing ourselves is an expression of our dignity, our sovereignty. As if having help is abnormal, some kind of flaw or a malfunction. "I can do it myself" is a milestone, a sign that a child is feeling a sense of mastery over his world. But for adults, "self-sufficiency" is embedded in notions of choice, liberty, and freedom for and from others. It is a discourse that is defective, one that presumes us to be entirely autonomous, independent beings and that giving or receiving help indicates either control or its absence. We don't want to need help, but being helped fits the facts of human life as we know it: we were born needing help and we end life needing help. The thought of a child or an elderly person suffering without the help they need makes us sad. But needing help in the middle part of our lives too often also seems to us sad. Why does this case present us with a special problem?

9. Founders Archives.

Our parents' goal was that we would grow up and be "productive members of society." But not everyone can produce something with economic value. Rafi cannot provide a good or service. He lacks financial, social, or labor capital. In a world where efficiency is king, where our social worth is so often based on what we invent, accomplish, or achieve, the disabled present a unique challenge. And as such, the disabled are uniquely able to question and challenge these social values. The power to legitimize and acknowledge Rafi cannot come from commodification or productivity indicators. It comes straight from his humanity, as it should for us all. Rafi has value because human beings have value, and this value does not differ according to people's differences.

Rafi wants to belong. He wants to fit in, to be with people who treat him as normal and with respect. He can tell when someone is not comfortable. Yet most often Rafi does not belong. He is excluded as the world races by, as one unable to live according to the values of self-sufficiency, productivity, knowledge, and power. There are other values that must be agreed upon so we can discover his value, beauty, and uniqueness.

In this task, Jean Vanier offers us a vision we might follow: "We tend to reduce being human to acquiring knowledge, power, and social status. We have disregarded the heart, seeing it only as a symbol of weakness, the centre of sentimentality and emotion, instead of as a powerhouse of love that can reorient us from our self-centeredness, revealing to us and to others the basic beauty of humanity, empowering us to grow."[10]

This Book

This book is about difference: its inescapability, its joy, its challenges. You've already read a little about myself and my own process of learning to lean into difference. In the chapters that follow we will explore biblical approaches, issues of limitations and belonging, acceptance and lament, through different kinds of difference and disability. My reflection proceeds with this basic claim: Humans are characterized by being both created in the image of God and different, and that a concern for difference remains central to God's heart. God is deeply implicated in human difference.

Before we plunge in, a word about one part of my own difference is in order here. I am both Jewish and Christian, and I write as one steeped in both those traditions. For some people that's an impossible combination

---

10. Vanier, *Becoming Human*, 55.

and for others that can be harmonious. I am Jewish and I assert that Jesus is the Messiah of Israel and the Savior of the world. He is the fulfillment of the hope and destiny of Israel and her civilization.

You may not be comfortable with the references to God and the Bible and Jesus, but those form the foundation of my thought. I hope you will still be willing to follow that conversation. You are welcome here. I draw comfort for Rafi and for myself from these texts and from our shared humanity with those who have gone before and wrestled with God.

Workbook Questions

1. Consider the opening epigraph about Jewish prayer. What is the difference between the two blessings and why might they be appropriate for two different situations?

2. What has been your own most profound experience of difference, that forced you to rethink some of your assumptions?

3. Can you think about some of the ways that you consciously and unconsciously isolate and protect yourself from difference?

4. "The thought of a child or an elderly person suffering without the help they need makes us sad. But needing help in the middle part of our lives too often also seems to us sad." Why is this, and what does it tell us about our assumptions and expectations?

2

Difference and the Body

I REMEMBER THE DAYS after he was born, I kept looking at him. I really did not see it. Denial, I guess. We were still waiting for the genetic testing to come back, but the doctor showed us clearly his neck and his eyes, nose, and the crease on his palm. That was how he came to the diagnosis. Rafi has almond-shaped eyes that slant up and a short neck. A flattened face, particularly the bridge of his nose. He has a small stature and a single deep crease across the center of his palm. You can say that Rafi's body is different, but you cannot say this is a good thing or bad thing. We have been taking care of Rafi's body for twenty-six years. His body requires more maintenance than some, less than others. He sees all kinds of specialists to help with his body: ears, heart, eyes, teeth, gums, nose, bones and joints, feet, skin. He has seen three psychiatrists, several speech therapists, psychologists, occupational therapists. We had two girls after Rafi. The amount of work for each was different. Different is normal.

Our Body and Our Humanity

Something extreme happened to Robert McCrum's body. When he was a young and vigorous newlywed, a sudden stroke left him unable to use his left leg and arm, and one side of his face had become frozen. He explains, "I was not in pain, but I was oppressed with an overwhelming fatigue. The smallest thing wanted me to lie down and go to sleep . . . [S]itting in a chair . . . was exhausting."[1] Eventually, when McCrum was released home from the hospital he would measure the time it took him to perform simple tasks. "Six months ago I could slip across the street to post a letter in the time it takes to type this sentence."[2] But following the stroke these routine tasks took him much, much longer. This realization taught him something about his limitations: "I am acutely reminded that there is a world out there, a world I cannot be part of in quite the same way." But another side effect of his stroke has been a new and more casual approach to the stresses and worries of the world. He now thinks "so what."[3] His new dependence on his wife created a vulnerable intimacy for which he is thankful. "I have become friends with slowness both as a concept and as a way of Life."[4] His body and its relationship to the world and to time has changed forever. His body is now different.

What Is the Body?

Some of our biggest problems come from how we and others see our bodies. But we do not "have bodies"—we are bodies. It is only through bodies that we come to be. Bodily existence is an essential part of being human and all human experience is mediated through our bodies. To be human is to exist in a body.[5]

Rafi's body is central to how he experiences the world, not just an empty container. His body means something. Rafi also uses his body to get at the world. The way he gets at it is just his own. There is no "normal" here. We know what it is to live in a body and that our differences are sometimes obvious and sometimes less so. Our bodies—Rafi's, yours, mine—are vehicles for doing God's work in the world, ones that theologian Ephraim Radner calls "tools of grace."[6]

In this chapter I want to think critically about Rafi's body and our humanness. These are questions I have: What is the meaning of having a body? What is the meaning of Rafi's body? Does the outward difference

1. McCrum, "Lives," 116.
2. McCrum, "Lives," 118.
3. McCrum, "Lives," 118.
4. McCrum, "Lives," 118.
5. Radner, "Psychedelic Body." This is a very helpful personal and theological reflection on Hebrews 10:5.
6. Radner, "Psychedelic Body."

in his body make a difference? What is his body for and how should his body be used? I struggle to understand difference in ability and disability and normalcy. The more important question is what it means to be human. Quite clearly at a deep level, we are all different. Difference is the norm for human beings. If that is so, we need to think deeply about the language of difference and living with difference.

Sometimes people speak with all good intention about "healing our differences." I wonder where Rafi would disappear to without his difference. How would I recognize him? How would we recognize each other without our differences?

Wondering about the body has an impressive history in philosophy. What kind of thing we are breaks down into two major views: Dualism asserts we are a body and something else. Some combination of material and immaterial, or body and soul. In contrast, monism claims that we are just a body. Just one thing but a specific kind of thing.

Both positions agree that the body can do certain things: hope, sleep, fall in love, plan, scratch, reflect, write poetry, desire. So we generally agree that people are bodies that have particular abilities and characteristics, and difference from other things. It is these particular abilities make us human. Are we just bodies that fulfill functions? Rafi's body does pretty much what other bodies do, even if the pace and orientation of his body are different.

I am not sure what happens in Rafi's body. I do not know that he reflects much: evidence points to thinking mostly about his next meal. His body seems happy. He listens to music and his body dances, he laughs and his belly jiggles, he does yoga, lifts weights and shoots baskets and plays tennis. His body does all that. He smiles and frowns and laughs. He doesn't seem to be in pain. He expresses frustration, anxiety. It looks like he gets depressed now and then. Generally, he has an easy smile and seems content in his body.

Rafi's relationship to his body is pretty much like everyone else's body, but there seem to be social norms that work against this realization. His body cannot join in and participate with most of the ways that bodies do things together. Enormous accommodation would need to be made and the other bodies would feel that their bodily experiences were hindered. It's hard to integrate Rafi's particular body with what other bodies are doing. But this is not a matter of "good bodies" and "bad bodies." Have you watched an "able-bodied" person try to play wheelchair basketball? Suddenly it's not so clear who is different and who is normal.

Creation

According to the Genesis account, when God created man, he began with bodies: God formed the physical body first and only then did he breathe into them. The body is the central aspect of being created.[7] Adam and Eve walked and ate, drank and played. All that was an experience of the body. We are at least as much "ensouled" bodies as we are incarnated souls. This affirmation of physical existence opposes any notion that the body is inferior to the spirit. The body is presented as a gift, which evidences God's wisdom and power: our bodies are revelatory.

The biblical tradition speaks of it this way:

> I praise you because I am fearfully and wonderfully made; your works are wonderful, I know that full well. My frame was not hidden from you when I was made in the secret place, when I was woven together in the depths of the earth. Your eyes saw my unformed body; all the days ordained for me were written in your book before one of them came to be. Ps 139:14–16

Is Rafi's body fearfully and wonderfully made? His body is not an impediment to communion, service, or worship of God. The values of love, joy, peace, forbearance, kindness, goodness, faithfulness, gentleness, and self-control are all expressed through our bodies. Our bodies are able to do God's work. We cannot escape them: we must use them as they are given to us. While indeed some improvements can be made through discipline, decay and morbidity come to us all.

Rafi's body and its particular differences are how he interacts with creation, and this must be a form of grace, for him and for each of us. It is a blessing to have a body and through it we experience birth, family, struggles, pain, and hope. That is and must be sufficient.[8] It is all that Rafi has, and we must embrace it even if it does not resolve. What he does with his body is how he serves God and so in some way his body is his mission, so I hope he uses whatever kind he has, and that he and we are able to acknowledge it as a gift.

Spirit is framed by the body. The body is not just a container, it is a partner. The great hope Christians have of the resurrection places our bodies as the focus of destiny. The New Testament says that "we must all appear before the judgment seat of Christ, that each one may receive the things

7. Radner, "Psychedelic Body."
8. Radner, "Psychedelic Body."

done in the body" (2 Cor 5:10). God's ultimate endorsement of the physical body is found in the incarnation, where Jesus' body becomes the position for God's redemptive activity in the world.

Who Owns Our Body?

The modern world would assert that one's body is detached from anything but oneself, that it is sovereign. But all evidence from our lives suggests that this cannot be true. This certainly does not apply to Rafi. His body is his own, but it is guarded and cared for by many people. We want to say that our bodies are ours to do what we want with, but I think there is more to consider. The Bible maintains that God owns our bodies: "I praise you because I am fearfully and wonderfully made; your works are wonderful, I know that full well" (Ps 139). "For you were bought with a price. So, glorify God in your body" (1 Cor 6:20). The body is a sacred gift, and I am to relate to my body as a grateful steward rather than an autonomous owner. Our bodies can give and receive pleasure and pain to and from others. It is through our bodies that we can procreate as a means of carrying out God's creation mandate that we fill the earth and care for it, even if some—Rafi among them—cannot participate in that part of having a body. God loans us these bodies for the duration of our lives, and we return it to God when we die.

The Beautiful Body

To look at a social media feed one would think that life was a series of expensive and intense meals and activities with beautiful people who love and adore you, exotic and compelling vacations in magnificent places, empty beaches, and a constant stream of profound encounters. A beautiful body is an essential piece of the image and is only as far away as the next workout plan or diet discipline. What is a beautiful body? I do not know if that question can be answered, but we live in fear of difference and comparison, that our bodies will be found wanting. How do we decide who is beautiful and what is the proper body? In 2013, a Swiss charity created mannequins based on the bodies of disabled people in a bid to raise awareness that no one has a perfect body.[9]

---

9. See https://spd.org.sg/disability-in-fashion/.

No one's existence in a body ought to need justifying. Rafi's body is what it is and need not be compared. There is a sense of brokenness in all bodies while we yearn for perfection, but that yearning is for something else. C. S. Lewis knew that beauty evokes longing for that which stands behind the sunset, the painting, the poem, a longing that can only be fulfilled by the transcendent reality that is God. As he wrote, "We do not want merely to see beauty, though, God knows, that is beauty enough. We want something else which can hardly be put into words—to be united with the beauty we see, to pass into it, to receive it into ourselves, to bathe in it, to become part of it."[10]

Rafi was created in the image of God. That begs the question of what kind of God would do that. If we interpret Rafi's body as "not normal," then does that mean he has not been created in the image of God? Or perhaps that God created him mistakenly? Is Rafi a consequence of sin or distortion? Our bodies, and their particular differences, tell us something about God. "Disability reveals the God whom we worship to be quite different from our unreflective assumptions."[11]

To think rightly about the body is to think of our createdness, our dependence, our distinctiveness. It does not point to power or autonomy, notions that are toxic to disability. We have a gift, and we are invited into the world and into human community through our bodies.

Caring for Other(s) Bodies

Hospitality is first and foremost about caring for the bodily needs of others. It is no accident that "hospitality" and "hospital" share the same Latin root. We see many cases of it in the Hebrew Bible: Abraham invites three wanderers to rest while he brings them water and food (Gen 18:1–5), Job actively watches for strangers so he can take care of their needs (Job 31:32), Rahab offers hospitality and protection to the two spies when they come to spy out Jericho (Josh 2).

In the harsh conditions of the ancient Near East, hospitality was not merely a question of good manners but a matter of survival. There are moral implications of providing water and food to those traveling through the severe desert conditions. Biblical law specifically mandated hospitality toward the stranger who was to be made welcome just as "you were strangers

10. Lewis, "Weight of Glory," 12–13.
11. Swinton, "God We Worship," 277.

in a strange land" (Deut 10:19). Hospitality makes room for the stranger's body, the strange body, the foreign body. Heed the stranger's treatment because you know the feelings of a stranger, for you were strangers in the land of Egypt (Exod 23:9).

Leviticus 19 is the centerpiece for living well with others, others who are more—or less—different from ourselves:

- Do not curse the deaf or put a stumbling block in front of the blind but fear your God (v. 14).

- Do not do anything that endangers your neighbor's life. I am the Lord (v. 16).

- You shall love your neighbor as yourself: I am the Lord (v. 18).

- The foreigner residing among you must be treated as your native-born: I am the Lord your God (v. 34).

This is premised on a sleight-of-hand: Our forebears were enslaved in Egypt, but we are not and so we are implored to reach past the boundaries of self and become strangers and we take on the existential reality of the enslaved. Hospitality requires us to remember our own difference, and for our bodies to be in proximity to the bodies of the stranger and the different. This slows us down. We prefer safe investments with our bodies and a kind of limited liability policy. But loving the disabled and the stranger and the different is not safe: force yourself into proximity so your heart will be broken open.

Concluding Thoughts on Difference and the Body

We are left with what we have. We are part of a vulnerable human state, in which we can be exposed or endangered at any time. We will all weaken and die. We have been and will be dependent upon the generosity of others. The body that Calvin described as "unstable, defective, corruptible, fading, putrid, and pining" is also the body which C. S. Lewis said "we must accept and embrace . . . in all its glory and buffoonery."[12] We all have our bodies, gifted to us to use. They work, they fail, they hurt, they comfort. Our bodies are the place where we occupy the world. We are here and nowhere else. It is our starting point. We all have ordinary and extraordinary experiences and needs in conventional and nonconventional bodies.

12. Rigney, "C. S. Lewis."

When we think of human difference in the body, I think of all our particular needs for assistance: glasses, braces, wheelchairs, hearing aids. Headaches, cramps, ingrown toenails, blisters, stomach aches, fear, paranoia, tiredness are times of temporary disability and utterly normal. It is no accident that God chose to enter this world as a vulnerable baby, dependent on the care of others for all his needs. He could have come in strength and power, but someone changed the Son of God's diapers, fed him, and cared for his scrapes and bruises.

We all encounter the world through our bodies and the body is a source of knowledge, but none of us encounter the world the same way. There is no point in which we call our experience normal, and no single body represents humanness. There is a range of possibilities—not bad, just different. To be human is to be loved, but it also means that we are both distinct and dependent. Caring for the body of others and being cared for is part of what it means to be human. At one moment, my vocation is to care for Rafi and his vocation is to be cared for. Yet when he rubs Laura's back, it is Rafi who gives the care, and Laura who is cared for. We are all called to care and be cared for. Rafi is a gift, and this was the way he was invited into this world and into my life.

Workbook Questions

1. Think about your body, and its particularity. How is it different from that of your sibling, your best friend, your neighbor?

2. What are some of the ways you've found your own body to be wanting, imperfect, broken?

3. If we are created in God's image, what perhaps can our bodies—mine, yours, Rafi's—reveal to us about God?

4. "Hospitality makes room for the stranger's body, the strange body, the foreign body." Take a moment to reflect on this: on the challenge of hospitality and otherness.

3

Difference and Time

I HAD A FRIEND who really wanted to get married. It was 1995 and she was anxious: "I'm running out of time." When she finally met someone, we argued. I thought it was hasty, but she was adamant, with the result that our friendship became strained. In 2020 they divorced, after raising two kids together. "What a waste of time," she cried to me.

Once I took Rafi to the doctor with an ear infection at one of those walk-in clinics where they rotate people in and out quickly. That is what we all want: to be in and out quickly. We do not want to wait. I was pleased to find the waiting room was almost empty. I did not want to waste time. When the doctor walked in, he looked at Rafi and asked him to explain what was going on. "My ear hurts." The doctor did not even look at me. He wanted to talk to Rafi so his patient could explain his symptoms. Is it your left ear?—yes. Is it your right ear?—yes! Is it a sharp pain?—yes. Is it a dull pain—yes. Nonspecific pain? Yes? Do you have a fever—yes. The doctor seemed to know that echolalia—repeating the last thing the doctor said—is common for the intellectually disabled. After this went on for a few minutes I tried to break in with the information that would speed things up and make this more efficient. But the doctor stopped me: "Let me hear it from him—I have the time." The doctor took his temperature, looked at his ears and nose, and listened to his lungs. The doctor wrote a prescription. I was amazed and embarrassed when I realized we ended up in exactly the same place we would have had the doctor spoken to me about Rafi as if he were not in the room. Sure, we might have saved a few minutes. An extra five minutes spent, for dignity and respect. Did we waste time?

"What time is it, Rafi?" He looks at his watch and says three o'clock and he is correct. He reads the time correctly, but he is not oriented to it in a way that you or I might be. Rafi seems to have very little concept of time. He is in it like all of us, but his life is not ruled by it. His life is not governed by it or subject to it. He has accepted time and tries to play its rules, but this is the world he has found himself in.

Sabbath Time

Clocks are everywhere. We find ourselves chasing time, buying time, losing time, and killing time. We have appointments, assignments, responsibilities. The clock drives us, and we are under its authority most of our lives. Even on vacation we are ruled by it: airline and hotel schedules, reservations for this and that. Meeting friends for activities. Lying on the beach and looking at your watch and seeing that it is time for the next thing. We say that we are responsible for our time and we want to use it wisely. We enjoy spending it with people we love. Sometimes things are a waste of time. What exactly does that mean? We ascribe economic value to time.

One Friday in Jerusalem I stepped out of a meeting at lunchtime for a break. The street was bustling, noisy and raucous. Scooters and bicycles urgently criss-crossing the boisterous market, cars and buses packed with people holding groceries. Preparations for the Sabbath were in full gear.

I returned to my meeting. When we took a break again at about five the scene outside was almost apocalyptic: no people, no buses or cars. The market was closed. Things felt still and quiet. What had happened in those three hours? The physical space was the same, but time had changed it.

We live in a world governed by distinctions in time. That afternoon in Jerusalem people were rushing through time to get ready for a different time: Sabbath time—a time beyond time.

The biblical description of each of the first six days of creation all end with "and there was evening, and there was morning." The seventh day is the only one that does not conclude that way. It is not said of the seventh day that there was evening, and there was morning. Thus the seventh day gives the impression of being a kind of endless day, a time that was never meant to end.[1]

1. Robinson, *Sabbath*, 22–23.

The Sabbath is understood as a depiction of life in the garden of Eden. "Eden was a place separate from the rest of the world, and Adam and Eve were the gardeners. Eden was the model for what the entire world could become, and humanity was meant to be the vehicle to accomplish that."[2] The weekly Sabbath reminds us of a way back to life with God, to Eden, to a hope for the future. Jewish tradition also understands the Sabbath as a taste of the world to come.

Rabbi A. J. Heschel suggests that time makes us uncomfortable:

> In our understanding of time, which, being thingless and insubstantial; appears to us as if it had no reality. As a result, we suffer from a deeply rooted dread of time and stand aghast when compelled to look into its face . . . Shrinking, therefore, from facing time, we escape for shelter to things of space.[3]

For Heschel, the Sabbath manifests "holiness in time,"[4] a time set apart for connecting with God. Because time is the core of our lived existence, what is important is the way that we use time. Judaism sees life as the opportunity to sanctify time. The word *kadosh*—holy—is used for the first time at end of the story of creation. It is significant that it is applied to time: "God blessed the seventh day and made it holy." There is no reference in the record of creation to any object in space that would be endowed with this quality of holiness.

The Sabbath is a picture of timelessness, a time outside of time. For Rafi, at least, theologically speaking, every day is a kind of Sabbath. The past and the future are ambiguous at best. He is innocent and uncomplicated about it. He is in the garden. He is Adam.

Time Today

We use general words and phrases to refer to a specific time, place, or person in context. Using words like "now," "then," or "next week" does not make much sense for Rafi. When we ask Rafi to join the world's accounting of time, he gets confused and frustrated. So often we treat people like Rafi as if they experience time the same as others and he simply does not.

2. Robinson, *Sabbath*, 25.
3. Heschel, *Sabbath*, 5.
4. Heschel, *God in Search*, 417.

When we think about Rafi and time, we must think about the time we find ourselves in: time that drags when we are bored and speeds up when we are in love. Time that is also measured in ways our ancestors could not have imagined. Our lives are shaped by this kind of time.[5]

For our ancestors, schools, the church, or synagogue kept time. The life of the community was oriented around a holy timetable: times of prayer. Funerals and weddings. Holy days. Seasons and occasions dictated how time was used. Today we have push notifications, and this has fundamentally altered our experience of reality. The rhythms of life have changed so that everything is immediate, and we feel compelled to operate on this same timetable. We think we are getting more done in less time, but who decided we had to get this much done? This man-made time imposes something on us that feels distinctly less human.

As I think about this topic, I am struck at the obvious problem that time presents to Rafi. Rafi is considered delayed. Delayed compared to what?

What has gone wrong with our sense of time? It rules us as like a dictator. It is unrelenting. When we encounter people, we make social contracts, implicit agreements, about time and the way we use it, how we perceive it and expect things to happen. How much time do you have? Is this a good time? When does it open? When does it close? Are you worth my time?

We talk about family time, spiritual time, and leisure time. We have made it sacred and mechanized it. We are in love with speed, and we worship efficiency. When we think about all the pieces of our lives—family, work, leisure, study, private, date night, prayer, quiet—these are all things that are linked together by the clock. Our relationship with time and speed is seen as normal.

Creating and buying time, selling time, winning time, using time, saving time, wasting time. We measure it and create it and we insist on punctuality and synchronicity. These concepts of time make no sense in relation to Rafi. We want to be able to measure the exact location of past events. The commodification of time is a human construct and utterly strange to someone like Rafi. It does not exist, but we find ourselves in a world where to be mortal is to have your life tracked according to a rhythm that can be measured.

Some years ago, I was on an airplane that had just been outfitted with wireless connectivity. We passengers were all very excited. It was free for the time being as they were just beginning to equip their entire fleet. The

5. Swinton, "Lecture 2." This lecture has been invaluable to my thinking on this topic.

plane leveled off and we were cruising miles above the earth when the captain turned on the WiFi. It got very quiet, and the devices came out for our movies, emails, and FaceTime. It felt a bit miraculous. Suddenly we could be so much more efficient with our time. Imagine all we could achieve in these few hours.

As suddenly as it had appeared, the WiFi failed. The captain apologized, explaining that this new technology was still being worked out, and that we would have to manage without connectivity for the duration of the trip. Strangers began talking and griping. Partial flight refunds were discussed. It became a very social time. I enjoyed it more than the WiFi and wondered what it said about us: this marvel of an invention and its ingenuity, creativity and science that did not exist yesterday and then it did, and then when it did not work perfectly, we complained.

History and Cultural Obsessions

In the modern world, disability has become a handicap. The term originated in a seventeenth century gambling game where money was drawn from a hat—if you lost then your odds improved in the next game, a term that migrated in the eighteenth century to horse racing and the weights they wore. But it was only in the early twentieth century that it became a label used to refer to any kind of disadvantage or extra burden a person carried.

Life becomes a race, in which those who cannot compete are handicapped by being too slow. "Retarded" is a measure of speed, and the concept of developmentally "delayed' is based on evolutionary models and competitive economic races. What happens to those who can't keep up? And how did we come to construct this kind of normal in relation to time?

We have become obsessed with our own potential, seeing ourselves as self-created entities who can "be anything we want to be," based on our individual achievements. Happiness is tied to productivity, and this productive use of time is used to determine worth. As a result, the disabled and the different are vulnerable and they challenge the world and time.

Rafi, by definition, is locked out of this kind of society, where disability and not achieving goals "on time" becomes a liability to the march of progress. The way that the disabled use their time is incompatible with industrial, commodified time. Access-based disability studies often seek to return a sense of productivity to the disabled: how can you be happy or fulfilled if you cannot produce anything?

The label "disabled" is used to indicate those whom we must work to fix, and in fixing, to reassemble back into a time of efficiency and production. As Henri-Jacques Stiker notes in *A History of Disability*:

> The "thing" has been designated, defined, framed. Now it has to be scrutinized, pinpointed, dealt with. People with "it" make up a marked group, a social entity [. . .]. The disabled, henceforth of all kinds, are established as a category to be reintegrated and thus to be rehabilitated. Paradoxically, they are designated in order to be made to disappear, they are spoken in order to be silenced.[6]

I want to think critically about time and human difference, and Rafi. People who are different share time with us, and different people are affected by time in different ways. What do we do about time when we are in proximity to human difference and disability? When we are in proximity to the disabled, time is different. How we ask people to accommodate to that is foundational to our thinking about inclusion and belonging.

In *Touching the Rock*, John Hull wrote about his own experience of blindness. His is a story of how different bodies encounter the world differently, and one in which he learned to develop a new relationship with the physical world and with time. For Hull, time became slower, more condensed and controlled. His world became smaller. Hull mentions the particular experience of time of his friend Chris, who has multiple sclerosis. For Chris, Hull writes, "Time . . . has strangely expanded. It takes him 45 minutes to tie up his shoelaces in the morning. It doesn't matter. He does not get impatient. He just does it. This is how long it takes to tie his shoelaces."[7] As Hull discovers, things do not take time. Rather, our bodies take time and ultimately time takes our bodies. There is no such thing as long or short.

How do people with the difference of disability experience time? What does this difference mean? I want to understand what time is for, how we are meant to use it. Disability and difference have implications for our understandings about time and how it is used; it draws our attention to the nature and power of time. We see more clearly the way in which it is distorted and wrongly conceived of. Time must be reckoned differently when you consider the experience of people who are different and disabled. Disabled bodies force us to think about God's time in contrast to a modern industrialized clock time, which is commodified and utilitarian. God's time

6. Stiker, *History of Disability*, 133–34.
7. Hull, *Touching the Rock*, 79–80.

seems slower and more focused, as does disabled time. Rafi has all the time in the world.

God's Time

In *The Gift of the Jews,* Thomas Cahill asserts that the Hebrew Bible changed history by creating history. Because this God, unlike every god before, "cannot be manipulated." He is "a real personality who has intervened in real history, changing its course and robbing it of predictability."[8] Thus Cahill asserts that the gift of the Jewish people is time: time that is connected to human freedom and dignity. We are not slaves to a ruler, human or otherwise, rather we can make decisions about how we use time.

Time, as all creation, was created good. But somewhere it too became broken. The New Testament indicates that it is Jesus who redeems time, taking fallen time and using it for godly purposes. God enters into time, into our history, into our woe and sickness and slavery, to make time for us. Disability draws attention to the fallenness of time and helps us to understand what it means to reimagine and redeem it. Being obsessed with time will ultimately make us sad and anxious. In time the able body is mortal and in due course we are all disabled. Time wins.

Rafi has little awareness of time and history. He sometimes remembers his mistakes and tries not to repeat them, but the normal burden of memory does not seem to be present for him. Rafi is not a person of the past or even of the future but of the immediate moment. He has no plans for tomorrow, even though we write a schedule for the next day as this seems to bring him comfort. Whether those plans correspond to reality does not seem to matter too much. He has no autonomy or the capacity to lead his life autonomously so he cannot really plan.

In my efforts to make sense of God's time, I think about Paul's language of being in Christ. For Paul, all we are exists in Christ. As he writes in Colossians, we are hidden in Christ. Our autobiography is there. Who we are is already "in Christ." The notion of all being "in Christ" can help us to think differently about time, space, and possibilities.

Strikingly, Jesus said, "come to me all who are weary, and I will give you rest" (Matt 11:28). This envisions how we should relate to disability: disability helps to remind us of what that might look like. Time like this is entirely a gift because all things are made by God, are given by God to us,

8. Prager, "Gift."

including our selves. Time is something that we are to use as a gift, out of this gift.

My friend Ephraim Radner is a professor at Wycliffe College at the University of Toronto. He has written and thought a lot about time.[9] Ephraim has spent some time with Rafi, so I asked him about all this. His response was illuminating. He explained to me that Rafi's time is a window into the mysterious giftedness of all things that we frequently obscure by submitting creation to a few limited "uses" (getting things done, production, goal-achievement of one kind or another). That is to say that Rafi's time stands on the same plane as other uses of time, even if it is not directed at "usefulness" the way that so many of us direct our time. Many of us, I assume, will share Rafi's experience of temporality only at our deaths, that is, as we die.[10]

People with disabilities do not cry out for power or success; their energies are used for seeking out the warmth of relationships. I notice how many of us able-bodied folks have our eye on the clock, mindful of our next meeting, a talk to give, people and deadlines to meet. Rafi is not controlled by time in that way. He is, like so many with disabilities, fully in the present, "sometimes enjoying themselves, sometimes angry, usually trusting in the presence of people who appreciate them."[11]

C. S. Lewis suggests that we naturally assume that our own particular sense of time is more than just an experience, but is actually the way that things are structured:

> We tend to think of our experience of time as exactly equivalent to the ultimate nature of time. This assumption implies in turn that God interacts with time in the same way that we do—that His divine life is, like ours, a series of moments, and one moment disappears before the next comes along: and there is room for very little in each . . .You and I tend to take for granted that this Time series—this arrangement of past, present, and future—is not simply the way these things come to us but the way all things really exist.[12]

In Narnia, Lewis sees true hope in reoriented time: "Do not look so sad. We will meet again soon." "Please, Aslan," said Lucy, "what do you call

---

9. See Radner, *Time and the Word*.

10. Personal correspondence with Radner, June 22, 2020.

11. Vanier, *Becoming Human*, 67.

12. Lewis, *Mere Christianity*, 138.

soon?" "I call all times soon," said Aslan; and instantly he was vanished away, and Lucy was alone.[13] For Lewis, Aslan is not limited by any frame of reference or the speed of light, so that he can simultaneously encompass all other frames of reference. In *The Screwtape Letters* Lewis expresses the point of our desire to live in redeemed time:

> The humans live in time but our Enemy [God] destines them to eternity. He, therefore, I believe, wants them to attend chiefly to two things, to eternity itself, and that point in time which they call the Present. For the Present is the point at which Time touches eternity. Of the present moment, and of it only, humans have an experience analogous to the experience which our Enemy has of reality as a whole; in it alone freedom and actuality are offered them.[14]

Surprisingly, then, Lewis says that eternity is most closely related to the present: "The future is, of all things, the thing least like eternity. It is the most completely temporal part of time—for the past is frozen and no longer flows and the present is all lit up with eternal rays.[15]

When I think about God and time, I think of how he loves, waits, and rests. Scripture says that God acts "in the fullness of time," which I take to mean that love takes time. Disability time is slow time. Disability time is remaining in the present moment. Disability time is a comfort with waiting. This seems rather reminiscent of God's time.

Concluding Thoughts on Difference and Time

When we think of normal time and disabled time, we might notice the similarity to comparing industrial time with God's time. The slowness of disability is close to the heart of God, but God is also with those who move quickly; it is just different. Each body holds its own time, and each task is completed by timelessness not efficiency.

Accompanying people with disabilities requires slowing down. Unfortunately, today this gift is reversed into a charity or employment for assistants. We give the disabled our time in charity, relief, and support. The person with them is a worker who is paid but becoming friends with disability is learning how to receive.

---

13. Lewis, *Dawn Treader*, 162.
14. Lewis, *Screwtape Letters*, 228.
15. Lewis, *Screwtape Letters*, 78.

How can Rafi have friends? He forms friendships differently because of time. Stanley Hauerwas reflects provocatively on time when he says:

> The movement that Jesus begins is constituted by people who believe that they have all the time in the world, made possible by God's patience, to challenge the world's impatient violence by cross and resurrection.[16]

I struggle to have all the time in the world to be in proximity to Rafi, which is a challenge to the world's impatience.

Slow time gives us the space and the opportunity to be gentle, as Jesus himself is (Matt 11:29). Gentleness is also a fruit of the Spirit (Gal 5:22–23), and believers are commanded to be gentle (Eph 4:2). Here we can see what time is and what it is truly for. Our lives cannot be defined by production and usefulness. God's time both contains gentleness and is gentleness. Disabled time is gentle time.[17]

I think that God is deeply embedded in all of this: in disability and difference and in time. Love takes time and is attentive. Clock time is a life of individuality. Community time is different time. Efficiency, contribution, autonomy is high-speed time. True proximity demands time. Slowing down makes space for difference. We all yearn for deeper and truer connection: with one another, with our deepest selves, with God. But our hyper-efficient and hyper-cognitive commodity culture works against this ability to make unhurried time for the other. We need proximity and this proximity takes time. It slows us down. Slowness can be a gift and we must start reorienting ourselves to outcome and not speed, and to taking the time to be fully present with those who experience time differently.

When you are in proximity to difference and disability you find different patterns of knowing, loving, and time. Time stops being anxious. The giving of time and the receiving of time is different. It is counterintuitive—inaction becomes advantageous. The concepts that we understand as achieving and losing changes meaning. Time becomes dignified under God's command.

16. Hauerwas, *Matthew*, 37.

17. Swinton, "Disability, Time, Spiritual Dimension."

Workbook Questions

1. Consider the opening story of Rafi at the walk-in clinic. Have you ever had a realization like the one that the author had, in terms of thinking differently about time and efficiency?

2. Think about your own relationship to time. How are you enslaved to time? How do you keep time? How do you "waste" time? What is time "well-spent"?

3. "Disabled bodies force us to think about God's time in contrast to a modern industrialized clock time, which is commodified and utilitarian." Are there other kinds of bodies, or aspects our own bodies, that might help us to enter into God's time?

4

Belonging, Including, and Hospitality

WHERE DOES RAFI BELONG and where is he included? Where does he go? What is his place? For the first years he was cared for like any other small child. When his sisters came along and our house was busy, Rafi just fit in as the older brother. With Rafi there were lots of doctors to be visited, forms to be completed. We started the advocacy process, but everything still seemed like a fight when it came to his belonging in school. There were lots of services and organizations, but it was a labyrinth and we had trouble navigating it.

I remember endless meetings with school officials who too often treated us like we did not full appreciate the challenges. Sentences that began with "you have to understand . . ." It was all about inclusions and resources and unions. But we were blessed with some wonderful teaching assistants and Rafi made his way through elementary and middle school. Many people knew him—he is charming. It was obvious, however, that Rafi did not fully belong.

The decision to segregate him was a hard one. We had hoped for him to be integrated into public school where his presence would serve as a testimony and a demonstration, but it was simply too difficult. We reluctantly decided to put him into a high school that was just for people with special needs. It was an amazing school with some very profoundly different people and a large, caring staff. Those were good years for Rafi and he found a place for himself in this high school. It was a place where he belonged, but he did not have any real friends.

Most people who have children with Down syndrome are older parents who have had unexpected pregnancies. The parents we knew of were much older and obviously bewildered and struggling. We found no real fellowship in professional or personal associations. We were younger parents and Rafi was our first child, without any outside supports beyond what we paid for. The problem of belonging did not only affect Rafi, it affected us as his caretakers too.

Including and Belonging

I have spent a lot of time not really belonging, as a stranger in the houses of strangers. I often traveled from place to place speaking in local churches and would stay overnight. In advance of the meeting, arrangements were discussed and decided. Arrival time, housing, meals, and other logistics. I did this for thirty-eight years. I think that being a stranger and being disabled have something in common—a vulnerability and a sense of a forfeited or lost identity. Lack of status. Estrangement. Dependence on others.

Rafi is vulnerable. The sojourner is vulnerable. It is a different type, but the weakness and helplessness are still there. The sojourner's vulnerability and dependence is addressed in the Hebrew Bible through the repeated portrayal of the sojourner as special recipient of God's favor, protections, and benevolence.[1] The typical sojourner is aware of it, Rafi is not.

When it comes to hospitality for Rafi, there is intentional effort and planning required on both sides. Traveling with Rafi is challenging. There is risk that things will be out of sorts and that Rafi will make a bit of a mess. Hosts must be flexible and open to difference. Rafi is aware when people are truly welcoming and hospitable, and he is uncomfortable in contexts where his difference is not met with contentment and ease.

When you enter a home as a stranger, there are clear vulnerabilities on both sides. The host sets the tone, and the guest tries to read the signals. Pictures, furniture, books, and smells. You try to take it in and evaluate what kind of home this is. Is it warm and welcoming or sparse and fearful? As a stranger you are vulnerable, so you wait for the signals. The host is vulnerable too, trying to understand and extend trust to the person that they have opened their home to.

1. Santos, "Biblical Bases," 42.

In a discussion about what qualities make a good host, Minh Phan, the chef and owner of Porridge & Puffs, in Los Angeles, said, "Maybe it's generational, maybe it's cultural, but my parents taught me that you can be sad inside, but you have to be thoughtful and not let people take on those burdens . . . It's so deeply ingrained in me, and maybe that's what hospitality is."[2] When I am a stranger in a home that is offering hospitality, my burdens are lifted. "Hospitality is both invisible and formidable—it surrounds you. You can find it at a rest stop on the highway and miss it at the host stand of a fine-dining restaurant. You feel its presence, or you don't."[3] It is a sense of safety and well-being and connection. It is a feeling of belonging in a temporary setting.

"To belong one needs to be missed."[4] That is the difference between inclusion and belonging: we don't miss people who are included, we miss people who belong. Belonging is a powerful way of envisioning the world differently. While Rafi is included in many places, inclusion is not enough. "Inclusion" is used in a way that is toxic to Rafi and those others who are different like him. It is a kind of self-centeredness that takes the life of the other person into its own hands and tries to define it. It suits its own purposes and only includes people on its own terms.

The disabled are not simply "included" in creation. They belong to God's creation. I do not think that God could imagine creation without disabled people and so the question is, "How do the disabled and the different belong?"

We are naturally drawn to people like us and to people who please us. This makes sense. There are common interests and personalities. But left to ourselves, without the disabled, it is difficult to imagine missing them. How do we need Rafi? How do we include Rafi in such a way so that we do miss him? How do we include Rafi so that he belongs? To belong, we need to be missed. When we are missed, we belong.

Here is the problem for Rafi: If he can only participate by voluntary choice, based on rational autonomy,[5] then his access is curtailed, and his dependence on others relegates him to the private sphere. The definition of normalcy excludes Rafi because we presume and are preoccupied with this autonomy. Rafi does not exist in the categories that obsess the rest of us:

2. Rao, "What Is Hospitality?"
3. Rao, "What Is Hospitality?"
4. Swinton, "Many Bodies," 23.
5. See Reynolds, *Vulnerable Communion*, 77–107.

autonomous, free, and self-constructing. He cannot make his own decisions or "write his own life story." Inclusion and belonging are out of his hands.

For his criticism of the Nazi regime, Dietrich Bonhoeffer was banned by the Gestapo from preaching, teaching, and finally from speaking at all in public. Eventually he was arrested and charged with conspiracy in April 1943, for helping Jews escape to Switzerland. Bonhoeffer was also connected to an unsuccessful plot to assassinate Hitler. He languished in a series of prisons and concentration camps until he was executed at Flossenbürg on Hitler's orders, just three weeks before the liberation of the city. His writings, some published posthumously, are considered Christian classics.

In 1933 Bonhoeffer visited a community of disabled and people with epilepsy, called Bethel. This was Bonhoeffer's first experience of human difference in disability, and it became a site of revelation for him, provoking profound insight into the nature of human existence and our ultimate vulnerability and defenselessness. For Bonhoeffer, all human life had worth, and even the most profoundly different and disabled were of value. Recognizing that the value of human life is independent of the utility value of that life, Bonhoeffer became increasingly indignant over the Nazi euthanasia program and the elimination of disabled life. He began to see the default categories of health and sickness as ambiguous expressions being mobilized in the service of a new humanity, the Aryan superhuman, freed from the genetic corruption of the disabled.

Bethel, in contrast, was a place of belonging. Bonhoeffer was so impacted by the experience that he preached a sermon in 1934 at St. Paul's Church in London as a warning against disdain for disabled life.[6] There he envisioned a relationship of a shared bond between all human beings, where power or weakness were irrelevant, and of belonging to one another because of our shared humanity and because of our Christian understanding of belonging in Jesus. For Bonhoeffer being in Jesus is the fundamental ground of our belonging. This is "life together." For Bonhoeffer, "the exclusion of the weak and insignificant, the seemingly useless people, . . . may actually mean the exclusion of Christ."[7]

6. See Wannenwetsch, "My Strength," 372.
7. Bonhoeffer, *Life Together*, 38.

Hospitality and Purity

According to the Babylonian Talmud, "A Pharisee may not eat with an *am ha-aretz*" (Berakhot 43b). This rabbinic directive separates Pharisees from the common people at the table out of fear of contracting ritual impurity. While purity laws were commonly followed, not everyone did so with the same level of stringency. Religious sects at the time, such as the Pharisees, priests, and Essenes, would have made more strenuous effort than others to avoid contracting unnecessary impurity. The Pharisees were meticulous about eating, and did not, as a rule, eat with people who were less precise.

Jesus, however, ate with everyone, even common people. To enter a home and share a meal was a symbol of intimacy and hospitality. Jesus touched the sick and other unclean people and shared meals with those who did not observe ritual purity. His apparent lack of anxiety concerning his own impurity might have been seen as scandalous and anti-social, although there is much scholarly disagreement and debate surrounding this issue.

> While Jesus was having dinner at Matthew's house, many tax collectors and sinners came and ate with him and his disciples. When the Pharisees saw this, they asked his disciples, "Why does your teacher eat with tax collectors and sinners?" (Matt 9:10–11)

The Gospels present us with a vulnerable Jesus, a sojourner in need of hospitality. But beyond this, Jesus embodies hospitality toward others, welcoming all to share in the divine banquet. His is a love without boundaries, a love that does not ask by what right the beloved deserve welcome. A gift is given, the value of which cannot be measured according to conventional mechanisms of exchange based in self-interest or calculated outcomes.

Here the stranger is welcomed as a neighbor, recognized as kin with subversive effect. This disorients and overturns standards of value based on status, race, gender, religion. Jesus asks us to reevaluate what it means to have a household. Home is for giving way to others, making places of belonging for the stranger. The despised, the poor, the unclean, the sick, all are invited into the household of God.[8]

> Then one of the Pharisees invited Jesus to eat with him, and he entered the Pharisee's house and reclined at the table. When a sinful woman from that town learned that Jesus was dining there, she brought an alabaster jar of perfume. As she stood behind him at his feet weeping, she began to wet his feet with her tears. Then she

8. Reynolds, *Vulnerable Communion*, 240.

wiped them with her hair, kissed them and poured perfume on them. (Luke 7:36–38)

Who was this woman who dined with Jesus? Was she a Jewish prostitute? In all these events surrounding eating and hospitality Jesus reverses and overturns expectations about human difference. Jesus talks about surprise and striving to enter by the narrow gate. His prime targets are the presumptuous and those who feel sure of their place.

Belonging and Hospitality

Tom Reynolds is a colleague, a theologian, and a father. His son has Tourette's syndrome with additional diagnoses of Asperger's syndrome, bipolar disorder, and obsessive-compulsive disorder. Tom reflects deeply on all these in his book *Vulnerable Communion: A Theology of Disability and Hospitality*. It is essential reading for anyone interested in this topic: intense, thoughtful, and heartbreaking.

Reynolds reflects theologically on how Christians might be more welcoming, able to think and act more openly and generously toward disability and people who are different. Hospitality, however,

> means more than the courtesy of providing access points for those otherwise unable to enter and find their way. Hospitality involves actively welcoming and befriending the stranger—in this case, a person with disabilities—not as a spectacle, but as someone with inherent value, loved into being by God, created in the image of God, and thus having unique gifts to offer as a human being. Yet we are up against complex social forces and theological assumptions that make the task difficult.[9]

Reynolds reminds us that hospitality is not just about the social world and human beings making more inclusive spaces for one another. Hospitality is also a signpost, a reminder and metaphor of God's love for us. "For hospitality is a gift offered without preconditions and expectations, an emblem of openness to the other. Accordingly, it is through the practice of hospitality that we participate in God's inclusive embrace."[10]

For Reynolds, the theological essence of hospitality is that God blesses through the stranger. How so? In hospitality the center of gravity lies

9. Reynolds, *Vulnerable Communion*, 16.

10. Reynolds, *Vulnerable Communion*, 20.

neither in the home nor in the stranger, neither in host nor guest, but in the God of both who is discovered redemptively in the meeting—indeed, in the role reversal.

Scripture calls people to be persons in relationship to others. Belonging is when others care about your needs and whether or not they are being met. We are not simply lone individuals who might sink or swim, some with better fortune and others less. We are called to be holy together, as one, in Christ. Thus, hospitality is not a matter of kindness or decency, but rather it broadcasts a deep sense of the belonging of others. And others are, by definition, different. All others. Hospitality is "loving your neighbor as yourself."

When the different belong, that belonging is felt and experienced in the body. Our bodies are the place where we experience this hospitality and the place where we come to know the world. The core of this experience of hospitality is God, and Jesus is the ultimate sojourner in need of welcome in our families, homes, and hearts.

This is not an abstract concept or idea, it is a practice: something that God does as he includes. I cannot know he loves me by reading about it. I encounter love in my body as I am embraced by the experiences of the love of others in the bounds of welcome. We reveal the Word of God through the practices of hospitality.

It is good to know things. But cognitive knowledge is not necessary for the Holy Spirit to do its work. Knowing things is just one aspect of our life with God. Those who cannot know in this way are held and sustained by those who do. Those who do know things are sustained by those who do not. There are many ways of being a disciple and many ways of knowing.

Hospitality, Rafi, and the Call of Matthew (Luke 5:27–28)

Jesus calls Matthew and the response is one of immediate obedience. How is it possible that Matthew followed him without knowing anything? Was there information given in advance? Had Matthew met with Jesus previously? Why would Matthew follow without understanding what he was getting into? We know that Matthew already had a big job and other responsibilities. What about his commitments? Was there no interview, no passing along of information?

All that we have is Jesus' call and Matthew's response. The text is not interested in the reasons behind his decisions. According to Bonhoeffer,

> Levi leaves all that he has—but not because he thinks he might be
> doing something worthwhile, but simply for the sake of the call.
> Otherwise, he cannot follow in the steps of Jesus . . . When we are
> called to follow Christ, we are summoned to an exclusive attach-
> ment to his person.[11]

Rafi has no comprehensible plan for his life. He is not striving for
something. Jesus called Matthew to himself. Jesus calls Rafi to himself.
Not to an idea or creed or confession, but to himself. Over time, Matthew
learned and experienced things, and I am sure the same is true for Rafi,
however differently. What is shared is the center of the call, the source of
the hospitality. That center is Jesus.

Hospitality has to do with receiving an invitation and learning to
trust. Can a disabled person be included and belong practically and theologically? Yes—love is embodied and revealed in spirit in human action.
There is nothing inequitable about following without words and concepts.
Not being able to express yourself is not a handicap to God, only a difference. The disabled learn to love and trust as they encounter the body of
Christ. Knowledge is not a criterion for inclusion, rather, understanding
is a consequence of inclusion. This movement is what we call discipleship.

Hospitality, Vocation, and Time

I am asserting that for Rafi, God's time is central to his discipleship and
vocation. If Rafi is called, then Rafi's tasks take place in redeemed time. If
the body of Christ does not realize this, then we have buried that talent.
"God does not need our good works, but our neighbor does."[12] This is what
it means to be hospitable in time. God's work is done in time by all his
disciples regardless of difference. This is the power of vocation in everyday
life, to glorify God with those who are our neighbors. It is about serving
others whose vocation might be to be present and receive care.

> If you find yourself in a work by which you accomplish something
> good for God, or the holy, or yourself, but not for your neighbor
> alone, then you should know that that work is not a good work.
> For each one ought to live, speak, act, hear, suffer, and die in love
> and service for another, even for one's enemies, a husband for
> his wife and children, a wife for her husband, children for their

11. Bonhoeffer, *Cost of Discipleship*, 63.

12. Wingren and Rasmussen, *Luther on Vocation*, 10.

> parents, servants for their masters, masters for their servants,
> rulers for their subjects, and subjects for their rulers, so that one's
> hand, mouth, eye, foot, heart, and desire is for others; these are
> Christian works, good in nature.[13]

Our theological world is hyper-rational, and activity based. The idea that simply being is enough, runs counter-intuitive to modern utilitarian thinking. The different and disabled must be included in hospitality and discipleship and vocation. But what is the vocation of the disabled—what do they do with talents? They receive care. There is a blessing and power in doing nothing. I say that there is value in the simplicity of presence in a world ruled by clock-time and productivity.

This does not mean that Rafi and others who are like him have no capacity for care, as I believe that a proper way to define humanity is to say we are care. Caring is the primary way to comprehend human life. We could not live together without care. This fundamental approach sees care as the most vital distinction of being in the world.

There is nothing we must do to win grace or earn God's love. Like Matthew, we are called just to be with him and to follow him. He gives what we do not deserve, and we do not get what we do deserve. We must aspire to let some have as their vocation their presence. Their vocation is to be cared for and our vocation is to care.

These, like Rafi, are simply in the world and they remind us who we are as creatures and friends of God. Rafi's vocation is to be, and as such to remind us of the heart of grace in a way that can transform us: to teach us that receiving care is not a waste of resources. To impress upon us that a person's value does not decrease because there is no economic production.

Concluding Thoughts on Hospitality and Belonging

We naturally tend to be drawn towards and seek to invite the charming, the connected, and the beautiful to share in our lives, less often the ugly, the sick, or the different. Hospitality that forces us into closeness with a disabled or ill body can be challenging and uncomfortable. People love Rafi but I am sure they are glad he is not their child. I would probably think the same.

Much of our regular lives seems ugly: replete with daily struggles, problems, conflicts, and illness. We tend to want a place of hospitality

---

13. From Luther's *Adventspostille,* quoted in Wingren and Rasmussen, *Luther on Vocation,* 120.

where we can perform a kind of picture-perfect, controlled tidiness, where things are pretty and work smoothly. We so easily forget that God is present, with us, in all the reality and challenge and disability—we think he must be elsewhere.

> Hospitality as recognition of, accommodation for, and advocacy with people with disabilities is necessary for the church to be church. We are prone to hide from vulnerability, subsequently shunning it in others. . . . This is the paradox of hospitality: through receiving another the host in turn receives.[14]

We all need hospitality, we all need to belong. How can the different and the disabled host you? In any way they can. Hosting is enabling and empowering. I have seen Rafi host and he takes great joy and satisfaction in it. It is tempting to let the "more efficient" host and expect others, the less efficient, be our guests. But it is also our responsibility to receive hospitality from others, not just give it. In clock-time this might be uncomfortable. But in God's time it can be transformational.

I invite you, my readers, into proximity with the different and the disabled so your heart will be broken open. This cost has already borne: God sent the Son to a place of disability and difference, and it broke his heart. He gave everything and expected nothing. We receive everything and give nothing. This is all gift love, for in God there is no hunger or need to receive, but only the desire to give.

Rafi receives. What does he give? His presence. What does he need? He needs everything. There is no commodity in this relationship. When Jean Vanier started to live with the disabled, he came to realize, as did I,

> that our humanity is not rooted in our productivity or efficiency, but rather in our ability to love and to be loved . . . this is rooted in the truth of the Gospel: compassion, proximity to the weak, openness of heart.[15]

"It is not good for the man to be alone . . ." (Gen 2:18). This was the first thing ever that was not good. We are not created to be alone. We are creatures of dependence, of relationship, of care. Thusly we begin our lives and thusly we end them. We must learn to live that way in between.

We aspire to be one community with one body with many members (Rom 12:4–6). This is the definition of true belonging. No part is favored.

14. Reynolds, *Vulnerable Communion*, 247.
15. Jesuits of Canada, "Jesuits & Jean Vanier."

Strength is not favored. Beauty is not favored. Usefulness is not favored. Lewis reminds us that

> there are no ordinary people. . . . next to the Blessed Sacrament itself, your neighbor is the holiest object presented to your senses. He is holy in almost the same way, for in him also Christ the glorifier and the glorified, Glory Himself, is truly hidden.[16]

Workbook Questions

1. Think about three places/spaces/contexts/communities where you know you belong. Then think about what it might look like if within those places/spaces/contexts/communities you were "included" instead. How would it look and feel different?

2. If hospitality is a reminder that points us toward God's love for us, what might we learn from God's love for us about the right way to practice hospitality? Does God "include" us, or does he cause us to belong?

3. Can you think of situations where you've found it easier to give hospitality than to receive it, or ways in which you've been uncomfortable with others' hospitality? What might be at the root of that, and how might it help us to practice both giving and receiving hospitality better?

16. Lewis, "Weight of Glory," 19.

5

Difference and Limits

It was my first and—at the time—most overwhelming disappointment. I loved to play basketball. I had made the high school team. As we readied for the first game the coach sat me down and gave me the bad news: I was cut. My skill simply could not compensate for my size. I had already stopped growing, while my peers developed beyond what my own body was capable of. I was devastated.

When Rafi was younger, he tended to wander outside the house. One day, I was away, and while my wife was in the shower he took his younger sister and went to the park. Once he tried to run out to the street. It was the only time I spanked him. I was so upset and humiliated that I had done this. Rafi does not wander off anymore. He waits on the porch for his bus or his helpers, and when they come, he calls out to let us know he's leaving. He seems to know that's important and a limit.

When I think about Rafi's limits, I am thinking about ways that he is restricted. The things we have set bounds for. Rafi cannot go out alone. He cannot eat alone—his windpipe is a bit smaller than average, and he has a propensity to eat quickly and choke. He will not know physical intimacy or independence. He cannot handle money or make autonomous decisions.

Like us all, Rafi will have different and changing limits for the rest of his life.

Limits

To limit something implies setting a point or line that a person or thing cannot or may not transcend. We have a set of rules, in society, in families, in friendships, about what is reasonable behavior. These rules establish limits. Limits are built in, or agreed upon, to facilitate functional interdependence.

Deborah Beth Creamer develops what she calls "a limits model" in her thinking about disability. "The limits model begins with the notion of limits as a common, indeed quite unsurprising, aspect of being human. . . . [They] might even be considered an intrinsic element of being human."[1] Limits are not bad, harmful, or to be mourned. Rather, limits are a normal experience of everyday human life.

Being able to choose implies limits. It means you cannot and ought not do everything and anything. Limits and choices are built into us—they fit the facts. I have no romantic notions about Rafi's difference or his limits. They are profound and unusually restrictive. His difference makes him utterly vulnerable. And yet, limits are something that we all share. While Rafi's differences demand a specific kind of care not shared by most others, we all are all living the same journey of dependence and independence.

In the Beginning

In the beginning Adam was alone and there simply was no human difference. In this time he was alone, we read that Adam was "working" and "caring" and "eating." I imagine him discovering things new about himself, his limits, and difference in the world where he has found himself.

But something was not good. With time, Adam reached a limit of himself, a lack. He needed something. Something needed to be done to overcome the disappointment, the not-goodness, of this limit. What had been created thus far was not enough. Something was still not good. That something was another human. Difference. Eve was the same, but she was also different. When Adam saw that sameness and that difference, he was overjoyed. Neither Adam nor Eve is portrayed as being different apart from their specific maleness or femaleness. Human difference was good, provided by God to alleviate the not-goodness of man being alone.

The text does not describe maleness or femaleness but we know that being alone was not good. Aloneness was a limitation that needed suitable

1. Creamer, *Disability and Christian Theology*, 31–32.

help. The text then describes that this helper was to be the first woman and the first wife. Adam and Eve's unity is described as one flesh. Adam's experience of isolation gives us a vision of what it is to be human. He was initially alone, and it was not good. Adam's very body revealed that he was created for closeness with another. He was created so that he would, in due course, be in proximity to difference. And it was good.

Genesis 2 shows us the core of what a human body is. "Just as humans are necessarily embodied, they are also imperfect. The fact [is] that the creation and initial activity of humans in Eden entails process, development, and change."[2] There was no obvious physical impairment in either body, and it seems that Adam and Eve were busy doing bodily things: breathing, living, eating, and walking, working, caring, planting. They have bodies, they are bodies, and they are using their bodies to do their work and God's work. Yet I see no reason to imagine they had perfect bodies or enjoyed no limits on what they could do with their bodies. It is a mistake to imagine Adam and Eve as Platonic prototypes of humanity—paradigms of perfection. Perfection implies uniformity and stasis. But bodies are both varied and variable. They are complex and subject to development and change.

Creation reminds us that we are embodied and dependent on others who have bodies. Rafi is no different this way. Our bodies define our limits. Our relationships are dependent on these limits. Denying our bodies or our limits denies God who made them. God invests himself in our bodies and in our differences, and it is through that human difference that we can thrive, procreate, have companionship, and partner with others. Aloneness is lack of completion, a lack that can only be filled by an other. The new partnership occurs because something is not right. That something is solitude. That isolation was a limit that needs to be overcome. "Without human variety, what are we to make of our relationships—variety makes them possible."[3] Adam needed a relationship. And for that, he needed difference.

It is not good for humans to be alone. Difference must emerge because vulnerability and interdependence lie at the center of what it means to be human. God's presence is not the solution to the problem of human aloneness. Instead, Adam needs Eve; people need other people. And other people are different, by definition. Humans need difference. Rafi needs me and I need him. He needs to be cared for and I need to care for him.

---

2. Estes, "Imperfection in Paradise," 9. I am indebted to his thinking on this topic for this chapter.

3. Reynolds, *Vulnerable Communion*, 182.

Within this original partnership of difference, the couple is given limits. We might think of the tree of knowledge as a symbol, representing the necessary presence of boundaries and signaling the possibility and potential of development, within limits.

We understand limits intuitively. We experience them every day. We use them and accept them:

> Opportunities arise from limits and from opportunities. Architects find inspiration from the limits of time, money, space, materials, and purpose imposed by the client. Painters find creative expression by accepting the limits of the media with which they choose to work, beginning with the limitations of representing three-dimensional space on a two-dimensional canvas. Writers find brilliance when they face page and word limits. All good work respects God's limits. . . . [T]he art of living as God's image-bearers . . . [is] to be found in observing the limits set by God that are evident in his creation.[4]

Human embodiment and differentiation require limitation, which in turn create the possibility for human love. Thomas Reynolds stresses this point: "Differences are good and blessed, the stuff of relationships. Alone we are incomplete; we need each other to be whole."[5]

Bonhoeffer reflects on this paradox of difference:

> This becoming one is never the fusion of the two, the abolition of their creatureliness as individuals. It is the utmost possible realization of their belonging to one another, which is based directly upon the fact that they are different from one another.[6]

Limitations and boundaries are not the product of sin or error. They are not unfortunate aspects of our humanity that we must learn to simply bear or strive to overcome. Rather, limitation is built into who we are from the beginning and is thus essential to what it means to be human.

> There is knowledge of the other person as a creature of God, and knowledge of the other person as simply the other person who stands next to me, limiting me; there is at the same time the knowledge that the other person derives from me, from my life and therefore there is love of the other person and being loved by him because he is a piece of me. All these things are to Adam the

4. Schmutzer and Mathews, "Genesis 1–11."

5. Reynolds, *Vulnerable Communion*, 182.

6. Bonhoeffer, *Creation and Fall*, 65.

bodily representation of the limit which is to make the limit easier to bear; which will enable him to bear it in love. The other person is the limit placed upon me by God. I love this limit and I shall not transgress it because of my love.[7]

There is an irony of unity and difference in the story that establishes the possibility for intimacy. This difference produces natural limits that are inside the structural design of the relationship: "The creation of the other imposes limits on us, but these limits, far from being negative, entail the positive corollary of human differentiation and the necessary ground for human love."[8]

Limits are not a concern, but rather a cause for celebration because,

> In his unfathomable mercy the Creator knew that this creaturely, free life can only be borne in limitation if it is loved, and out of this mercy he created a companion for man who must be at once the embodiment of Adam's limit and the object of his love.[9]

Genesis shows us that limitations and boundaries can have positive consequences, in the form of human difference, relationship, and interdependence. Limits existed before sin and are needed for us to live together, care for each other, and be accountable for one another; this is our vocation.[10] We are limited to our bodies. We are limited by the fact that we experience change and development and experience pain and loss. And we are limited by the presence of the "other," who calls into question our autonomy and self-sufficiency. Noticing the ways humans experience limitation opens up rich avenues for exploring disability theologically and for rereading biblical texts, such as Genesis 2, with and for those with disabilities. Without limits we would be subject to endless illusions about our own power and abilities. Human difference necessarily brings with it human limits, and these limits are embodied differently. The presence of limits is from God. It is good and it is inherently human. It is also undoubtedly difficult.

---

7. Bonhoeffer, *Creation and Fall*, 66.

8. Estes, "Imperfection in Paradise," 18.

9. Bonhoeffer, *Creation and Fall*, 66.

10. Estes, "Imperfection in Paradise," 19.

Rafi and Limits

When I spend time with Rafi's peers at his vocational center, I come face to face with the difficult enormity of human limits and difference. Some of it is heartbreaking. I cannot stop thinking of the young man who must wear a helmet because he strikes himself, of the young woman who makes high-pitched, cat-like noises. How do their families cope with this vulnerability and limitation day after day?

These people are severely limited and dependent. But my proximity to them also makes me more human. I am forced to consider my own mortality and my own limitations. "Our support for those who are people with disabilities and the acceptance of the explicit reality of our own limitations are not mutually exclusive activities but are, in fact, deeply related and connected."[11]

Rafi's difference compels us to think about our mutual dependence. Hauerwas is right in that "Dependence upon others is often deemed a moral, developmental, or biological failure, a passivity denigrating human life. We come to regret limitations and weaknesses, and indeed often view them in terms of being victimized by powers not of our own making."[12]

Moltmann agrees that:

> There is no differentiation between the healthy and those with disabilities. For every human life has its limitations, vulnerabilities, and weaknesses. We are born needy, and we die helpless. It is only the ideals of health of a society of the strong which condemn a part of humanity to being "disabled."[13]

When we minimize attention to human limits and difference, we become restricted to the consensus of the majority or to the interests and agendas of those in positions of influence and power. There emerges a cult of normalcy. It excludes those who are outside of that normal.

We are finite beings, and so, by definition, we are bounded. There are many limiting forces that operate on us. We all encounter limits, our own and those of others, and we all must live with them personally. I must bear with Rafi's limits, and my own limits, every day.

11. Block, *Copious Hosting*, 36.

12. Hauerwas, "Community and Diversity," 40.

13. Moltmann, "Liberate Yourselves," 110.

[We know] that these limits differ, and that these limits are accepted, rejected, accentuated, complicated, degraded, and lived in many different ways. It offers us the ability to think of the presence of limits as a natural and good aspect of being human that at the same time is inherently difficult and challenging. It provides us with a new paradigm to make sense of ability and disability. This perspective of limits does not universalize, relativize, or minimize individual experiences but instead proposes an area of common ground in the midst of the recognition of exceptional incarnated and environmental differences. It gives us a place for some very important conversations to begin. It does not dismiss the insights of the medical or minority models but offers a needed theoretical perspective that helps make greater sense of "the experience of disability."[14]

It is crucial to accept that limits and difference are normal when we think of our bodies.

Jesus: Margins and Centers

Jesus makes space for the strangers and the outcast and the different—those who are on the margins, the limits of society, the sick, the lame, the unfortunate. Jesus embraced this paradox—not in normalcy or strength but in weakness and difference. Jesus spent his life on these margins. Jesus calls us to join him on the margins. To be a follower of Jesus, then, places one there, on the boundaries.

Jesus intentionally sought men and women from the margins so that he could bring them into a place of belonging and wholeness. Instead of bringing those on the margins into the center, Jesus changed the whole location of the center. Rather than moving from the margins of society to the center of society, the new "center" becomes located in Jesus himself, regardless of power, status, health, or ability. The margin joins the center.

Jesus was the center even though he lived and died a social outcast in a small corner of the Roman Empire. He and his people were despised by his government and threatened by authorities both religious and secular. He was not from the best neighborhood and there seemed nothing special about him. Perhaps he had a funny accent as well.

The margin is where we most effectively share our truths about limits and difference. This is a shared human narrative that opens us to

14. Creamer, *Disability and Christian Theology*, 32.

the possibility of vulnerability, brokenness, and accepting ambiguity in our differences and limits.

Our abilities and our health are temporary. Some limits are more extreme, but the presence and pervasiveness of difference and limits is essential to what it means to be human. It is not something that we have to conquer or get past or heal. There is no flawlessness in our embodiment. We must "start with the human variations of ability as the norm, and . . . build theory and theology from that starting place."[15]

Concluding Thoughts on Difference and Limits

We are not the first to struggle with this issue. The ancient writers of wisdom literature wrestled with limits, difference, and the truth of the human condition. We find ourselves, like them, eager to make sense of things but more than a bit baffled by it all:

> When I tried to gain wisdom and to observe the activity on earth—
> even though it prevents anyone from sleeping day or night then I
> discerned all that God has done: No one really comprehends what
> happens on earth. Despite all human efforts to discover it, no one
> can ever grasp it. Even if a wise person claimed that he understood
> he would not really comprehend it. (Eccl 8:16–17)

The complaint is that we might not really know what is going on, but we are going to be tested on it anyhow. Rafi bears a characteristic shared by all humanity—he has limits. These limits should not surprise us. They are intrinsic to our human condition, and we all need them.[16] Since these limits are common to us all, I do not accept the stigmatization of Rafi's limits while denying my own limits or calling them "normal." Let us not

> pretend that we do not experience increasing limits as we age, and
> even refuse to acknowledge the future limit of death. In these de-
> nials, we live a lie . . .We must attend to the values that we place on
> limits, including on people with visible and profound limits, and
> must challenge our notions of what it is to be normal.[17]

Being different and having limits means making choices. Our first parents chose, and Israel chose. God asks us to choose, and thus Israel was

15. Creamer, *Disability and Christian Theology*, 32.

16. Creamer, *Disability and Christian Theology*, 104.

17. Creamer, *Disability and Christian Theology*, 129.

called to a decision on limits. "See, I set before you today life and prosperity, death and destruction" (Deut 30:15). The heavens and earth would bear witness to this choice.[18]

Commenting on the unique ethical construction of seeing human difference in the stranger, Rabbi Jonathan Sacks proclaims this "the Hebrew Bible's single greatest and most counterintuitive contribution to ethics. God creates difference; therefore, it is in the one-who-is-different that we meet God."[19]

Finally, the psalmist understood the foundation that limits play in human flourishing,

> Blessed is the man who does not walk in the counsel of the wicked, or set foot on the path of sinners, or sit in the seat of mockers. But his delight is in the Law of the LORD, and on His law, he meditates day and night. He is like a tree planted by streams of water, yielding its fruit in season, whose leaf does not wither, and who prospers in all he does. (Ps 1:1–3)

Limits are a blessing and a curse. We hate them and we need them. We judge God and others on them. We judge ourselves. We expect to be judged by God. I want to be a person who is generous with difference and who accepts limits of all kinds as an expression of our humanity. I must become so because I live with it every day. These are bewildering times, where we reject both human limitation and human difference. Yet I am certain that God is deeply present in both.

Workbook Questions

1. Consider some ways that your own body is limited at this particular time. Can you name those limitations?

2. Imagine living a "limitless" life. What might be some of the advantages? What about the disadvantages?

3. Western society is broadly disdainful of the idea of limits. What might this tell us about Western society? What does this mean for the disabled?

18. Craigie, *Deuteronomy*, 365–66.
19. Sacks, *Dignity of Difference*, 59.

6

Lamenting Difference and Suffering

MY LIFE HAS BEEN mostly free from acute suffering. Before my father passed away, I had not been to a family funeral in twenty years. I have never spent a night in a hospital as a patient. I have never missed a meal. I am mostly free of physical pain. I am not sure that I really understand what suffering is. When I found out that Rafi had Down syndrome, I had a glimpse of something like it; a glimpse of what I eventually came to understand as the silence of God.

When I was home alone that night it was the deafening silence that hurt the most. It was a silence of forsakenness, of weakness and disappointment. I felt like I had received a massive blow to the head, to the stomach. More like a dream than reality. I wanted to stop breathing and wake up and rewind the clock. Each breath was hard. This was not my life. This was not my life.

Sam walked in when I was sitting outside the neonatal intensive care unit one day. He knew something firsthand about suffering and grief. One morning, as a young man, he awoke in a dumpster, an alcoholic. Now Sam sat down next to me and held my hand in silence for fifteen minutes. Then he left. That was it. And it was everything. That silence held more than all the other words of consolation that had been brought.

> Can God trust you like that, or are you still asking for a visible answer? God will give you the blessings you ask if you will not go any further without them; but His silence is the sign that He is

bringing you into a marvelous understanding of Himself . . . You will find that God has trusted you in the most intimate way possible, with an absolute silence . . . If God has given you a silence, praise Him . . . A wonderful thing about God's silence is that the contagion of His stillness gets into you and you become perfectly confident—'I know God has heard me.' His silence is the proof that He has. If Jesus Christ is bringing you into the understanding that prayer is for the glorifying of His Father, He will give you the first sign of His intimacy—silence.[1]

God takes pleasure in making himself best known in silence.

Rafi's relative comfort has come with a price. Many people of difference and disability have come before, living in suffering and quiet desperation. The disability services, benefits, and resources in the city where I live exist because of the suffering and advocacy of many people over many years. I have inherited all that advantage and well-being. Rafi suffers less because many have suffered before him.

In a curious and ironic way, I am called to care for and alleviate Rafi's suffering in this world. Given this great vocation I may have missed something foundational as I lament over Rafi's difference and dependence.

This chapter is a lament about silence. I am in good company.

Avoiding the Silence of Lament

Technological advances have enabled us to avoid pain and suffering in ways that our ancestors could not have imagined. This is not a bad thing, in itself.

It becomes a problem, however, when all suffering, pain, sacrifice, and hardship are to be avoided or alleviated. Even inconvenience seems like something our modern Western society races to save us from, so that we can access ever more goods and services without ever having to step out of our pajamas.

Have I made comfort into a God?

Modern technology has given us the illusion of a control over things which we do not actually possess. We need to understand that frustration, disappointment, and yes, suffering and pain, are the natural condition of all people so long as we are in this world. It is not some natural human right to be free from this. This is especially true for those of us who follow Christ, sharing in his humiliation and sufferings.

1. Chambers, "God's Silence."

Our avoidance of pain and our society's standard of a kind of easy, happy prosperity means that we are unable to appreciate the role and place of suffering. I want to support Rafi and myself and my family. I want to make their lives more comfortable. Less painful. But I do not want to concentrate my hopes and happiness on the things of the world. The world cannot satisfy, and it was never meant to. I am not called to a life of pleasure, of happiness, of ease, but to a life of radical commitment. How do I achieve this while I take care of Rafi?

We cannot allow our temporal prosperity to blind us to this truth. We cannot look to our lives for ultimate satisfaction. Our families will eventually disappoint. I guarantee it. The world will eventually disappoint and let us down. Our suffering and pain are not permanent—neither are our comforts and joys and pleasures. Jesus said in this world you shall have trouble but be of good cheer because I have overcome the world. He has overcome not to get us out of trouble, but to be with us in the midst of our trouble.

The glue that united Paul's life with the message he preached was his suffering as an apostle of Jesus. Paul's suffering was the vehicle through which the saving power of God, climactically revealed in Christ, was being made known in the world. Had Paul rejected this suffering, Paul would have been rejecting Christ. To identify with Paul in his suffering was a sure sign that one was being saved by the "foolishness" and "stumbling-block" of the cross.

All Christians will suffer in one way or another: if not outwardly, then inwardly, through the long slow battle with temptation or sickness, the agonizing anxieties of responsibilities for a family, the doubts and uncertainties that can accompany obedience and faith, and the conflicts with the world, our flesh, and the devil.

These sufferings, properly understood, are things to rejoice in—not casually or flippantly or superficially, but because they are signs that the present age is passing away, that the people of Jesus, the Messiah, are the children of the new age, and that birth pangs of this new age are being worked out in them.

I have a friend whose father does not speak to him. What was most shocking though was that his father refused to meet or acknowledge his firstborn grandson. From that harsh moment, my friend's understanding of suffering was sealed. I am in awe of his faithfulness and his courage and bravery. He would understand the silence, aloneness, and abandonment I am reflecting upon. In that moment he identified with the silence, aloneness, and abandonment of Jesus on the cross. And I want you to consider your own abandonment as well.

You may think that I suffer with an adult son with profound disabilities. Yet I have met many in the disability community with far more overwhelming problems, which leaves me feeling fortunate and blessed. Many of us have friends in other parts of the world who live on little and do not have access to the kind of resources we do.

At this point much of our suffering is anticipatory—what will happen to Rafi in the future? What will happen when Rafi is older? Who will take care of him? Will he be treated well? In many ways it is his potential suffering that causes me the most pain and is shrouded mostly in silence. I think that suffering is a kind of deep identification with this current and anticipated silence and loneliness of the flesh. Suffering is aloneness, abandonment, forsakenness, and darkness. Suffering is the realization that there is nothing we can do with it but endure it.

There is not a single person in the story of Scripture who is not met by difficult circumstance, sin, trouble. Yet they are, and we are, the bearer of God's purposes. This is how we understand our lives as part of God's story. At the end the hope for the world and hope for ourselves come together. Every tear is dried. We share in the struggle and anguish of human history where the cross is a sign of victory and our pain is there to tell us something. Ultimately my personal story must find a place where I meet God's story and those stories must find their intersection at the cross. We don't stop believing in God in pain, rather it is in pain that we are confronted with the kind of God we do believe in.

Lament and Silence in the Bible—Psalms

Lament directed at God is pervasive in the Hebrew Bible. The text of Psalms is genuine. It is unsentimental, honest, gritty. It is plausible. We accuse God. We honor his presence while we lay blame on him for leaving us like this. The relationship of God and his people is a difficult one. Lament comprises about 70 percent of the Psalms. This is probably the most real that prayer gets. There is a tradition of protest in the human condition. "When it comes to the safety and survival of others, the prophetic option is to argue rather than to obey."[2]

2. London, "Judging God," 18.

I like that. I do not think God minds being accused. He knows that we experience him as complicit in the arrangement. Our disorientation is real, and he needs to answer for it. So, we sit him down in the dock. I use this analogy from C. S. Lewis, who suggests that modern human beings, rather than seeing themselves as standing before God, prefer to place God on trial while acting as his judge. "The ancient man approached God . . . as the accused person approaches the judge. For modern man, the roles are reversed. . . . [I]f God should have a reasonable defense for being the god who permits war, poverty, and disease, he is ready to listen to it. The trial may end in God's acquittal. But the important thing is that man is on the bench and God is in the dock."[3]

If God is the ultimate reference point, then I can come to him. I can complain with the full range of emotions. We demand to know "why?" and "how long?" Why has God rejected (Ps 74:1), abandoned, or forgotten (Ps 44:24) his people? The writers ask repeatedly where God is (Ps 44) and why is he silent (Pss 13:1, 83:1, 109:1), begging that he not leave us alone (Ps 51:11). We meet here a counterintuitive joining of absence and presence: "I say to God my Rock, 'Why have you forgotten me?'" (Psalm 42:9), and "You are God my stronghold. Why have you rejected me?" (Psalm 43:2). We have a meeting of interrogation together with a vow of trust.

Often, we see the reflection of personal suffering, one that is not primarily related to an enemy, but rather a profound description of need. Lament is rooted in a relationship to God and the disappointment in God's seeming silence. "Save me, O God, for the waters have come up to my neck" (Psalm 69:1). "Hear me, Lord, and answer me, for I am poor and needy" (Psalm 86:1).

The psalms of lament offer faithful language with which we can express our hurt, brokenness, anger, and disappointment at what we experience and about the silence and absence that we feel from God at those times. But his silence does not indicate his absence. God tabernacles with us and takes pleasure in making his presence known in silence even among a distraught people. When I was in silence that awful night I first heard about Rafi's difference, all these truths overwhelmed me. No answers, just comfort. Hope. When I left my house that night to meet Rafi, I looked around the neighborhood. Nothing much had changed but everything was different.

---

3. Lewis, *God in the Dock*, 100.

Lamentation in the Bible

Lamentation is to cry aloud:

> Is any suffering like my suffering that was inflicted on me, that the
> Lord brought on me in the day of his fierce anger? From on high
> he sent fire, sent it down into my bones. He spread a net for my
> feet and turned me back. He made me desolate, faint all day long.
> (Lam 1)

What does Jeremiah presume here? That God is present. He has inflicted suffering, sent fire down into Jeremiah's bones, spread a net, turned him back, made him desolate. And somehow, in all this, Jeremiah retains the idea that "the Lord is righteous" (v. 18)

This chapter is an acrostic poem. Each verse begins with the letters of the Hebrew alphabet, from verse 1, which starts with the letter aleph, to verse 22, which begins with the letter taf. In other words: My grief is from A to Z, beginning to end, so deal with all of it, every detail, nothing is left out. Pay attention to it all and pay attention to every detail. Everything we feel, we need to get out from start to finish. For me, that was especially the pain and puzzlement of difference and disability. Lamentations focuses on God. We cannot just fix what makes us suffer. I cannot fix Rafi. He is not any more fixable than I am. To want to or try to fix Rafi is to demean him. There is no technique, medicine, or therapy. I must face it.

Ephraim Radner writes about this tendency to feel like things can be fixed in what he calls our

> culture of replaceability, the environing expectations that anything
> that is amiss can be restored . . . We know, that is, that some things
> are unfixable, irresolvable, and definitive, just the way they are.
> God is the God of both sides of this conflict . . .[4]

Radner does not seek to "repackage" this silence. Sometimes things simply do not get better, and we don't understand it and we can't fix it. "We cannot pretend otherwise, and we are left to lament in what God has given and still declare it all a gift."[5]

J. R. R. Tolkien says that "a divine 'punishment' is also a divine 'gift,' if accepted, since its object is ultimate blessing, and the supreme inventiveness of the Creator will make 'punishments' (that is changes of design) produce

4. Radner, "Divine Irreplaceability."
5. Radner, "Divine Irreplaceability."

a good not otherwise to be attained."[6] Somehow, we are left to worship this God on both sides. We lament suffering and we know that it too is a gift from which the creator will produce a good. As Tolkien reminds us,

> the pain is actually a gift for us through which we can be ennobled. It will, in the end, serve a good purpose, for God can turn even evil to good uses, although we may not perceive it thus while it is present.[7]

When I read Lamentations with Rafi in mind, I see that the acrostic form makes sure not anything is left out. You can go over it again but always there is an end, eventually you have covered the territory of your lament. Sorrow and suffering are not forever. There is either healing or death for all of us: When you are at A, you know that Z is there. The text says this: Let the tears flow but let them end.

Lament and Disappointment

Am I disappointed that Rafi has Down syndrome? That's a complicated question. What is disappointment, exactly? Maybe it is missing the place we want to get to: hopes, dreams, destinations, expectations. If we do not make it or get it, we are disappointed. We are disappointed if we don't get what we want, or we get what we don't want.

I see my peers with their own adult children. The comparisons are inevitable, but toxic. I do not doubt that they are thankful that they are not in the position I am.

They have their own pain, I am sure.

I don't know much about their silence and suffering. I know that those who have many yokes to bear do tend to relate to me and Rafi at a different place. Like a fellow soldier in battle. There is a camaraderie to silence. As we all lose parents or cope with aging parents and dementia these peers circle back to me and friendships pick up. "How is Rafi?" is a more common question I hear from these friends.

I think about this disappointment in relation to Paul. What was Paul's expectation? It was Spain:

> I long to see you; I do not want you to be unaware . . . that I planned many times to come to you (but have been prevented from doing

6. Carpenter and Tolkien, eds., *Letters of J. R. R. Tolkien,* 286.
7. Carpenter and Tolkien, eds., *Letters of J. R. R. Tolkien,* 286.

so until now). But now that there is no more place for me to work in these regions, and since I have been longing for many years to visit you, I plan to do so when I go to Spain. I hope to see you while passing through and to have you assist me on my journey there. (Rom 1:13; 15:23–24)

Paul greatly desired to get to Spain. That was his hope and expectation. He wrote this letter because he needed help and support and hospitality. Did he make it or was he defeated? I do not think we can know, but what we do know is "I have fought the good fight, I have finished the race, I have kept the faith" (2 Tim 4:7).

This is the acute theological question for us and for the disabled: "Can we trust God even if our most pressing needs are not met to our satisfaction?" How we respond determines if we bear fruit. Simply put, the world cannot ultimately satisfy. Any permanently settled or established happiness we all desire is withheld in this world. God refreshes us along the way, but he does not encourage us to call these things our home. Our joy is to be found in him.

"Who is the God we Worship?" is the piercing title of essay by John Swinton. C. S. Lewis pinpoints the matter, in writing on the death of his wife: "Not that I am in danger of ceasing to believe in God. The real danger is coming to believe such dreadful things about him. The conclusion I dread is not, 'So there is no God after all,' but, 'so this is what God is really like. Deceive yourself no longer.'"[8]

Who is this God? "He gives us just what is given and does not pretend that it's something else." It cannot be "exchanged" it cannot be re-invested; it cannot be improved upon; it can only be what it is."[9] As Job remarks "Shall we receive good at the hand of God, and shall we not receive evil?" (Job 2:10). And "Is it not from the mouth of the Highest that both calamities and good things come?" (Lam 3:38). These bold statements offer claims about suffering and hope, and ultimately can help us to stake out the grounds of hope amid disability.[10]

Scripture assumes it is so, and so do those who have come before. In 1562 John Calvin wrote of his own suffering: "God keeps me bound by my feet. . . . [I]t is difficult for me to creep from the bed to the table.

---

8. Lewis, *Grief Observed*, 5.

9. Radner, "Divine Irreplaceability."

10. Radner, "Divine Irreplaceability."

Today I preached. But I had to be carried to the church."[11] Calvin suffered greatly from a many physical ailments. He was confined to bed and had to be carried to church. Why did he endure? He tells us in the dedication to his commentary on 2 Thessalonians: "My ministry . . . is dearer to me than my own life."[12]

Rafi lives in an in-between time along with the rest of us—between death and life, anguish and faith, heartache and joy. I am waiting with him in eagerness. Caring for him is dearer than my own life.

Concluding Thoughts on Lamenting Difference

How do we accept sacrifice and suffering as part of everyday spirituality? Is it possible to measure success in reflecting on and interpreting our own suffering? Do we so enshrine personal happiness that our friends, family, and children do not see in us the kind of sacrificial and suffering love and tragic vulnerability that makes our faith real? Our text assumes trouble in this world. Be prepared for, become comfortable with trouble and failure, suffering and sacrifice.

As I navigate my life with Rafi, I try to have reasonable expectations. Am I preoccupied with bigger, faster, smarter, convenient? These all make us feel what we lack. I want to live like this: to accept and expect trouble, and to know that adversity and limitation are part of life. The ordinary matters. I want to live an ordinary life with an ordinary family who has an extraordinary man to take care of.

Amid all that, it really is okay for things to suck from time to time.

When a child is baptized into the Greek Orthodox Church, I'm told the priest touches the child with a cross, indicating that sooner or later this child will bear the cross himself. Our clues are abstract, but the person is concrete. The clues converge on him. Our story is his story. We look to the one on the cross. I would not believe any of it if it were not for the fact that he gave no finished answers. He experienced all of it: the disability, the ugliness, the pettiness, cruelties.

He came unto his own. He came.

11. Shepherd, "My Ministry."
12. Shepherd, "My Ministry."

Workbook Questions

1. If we can agree that suffering is neither intrinsically good nor intrinsically bad, what value or purpose might it have?

2. "Can we trust God even if our most pressing needs are not met to our satisfaction?" Why is this such an acute question for ourselves, and for the disabled?

3. What are some of the unmet needs in your own life? Try putting it into words by composing your own lament to God.

7

Disability and Difference in the Hebrew Bible

I GREW UP READING the Bible in Hebrew school. But as I would discover, my reading was censored. True enough, Abraham, Isaac, and Jacob were the patriarchs, the heroes of my people. They threw off the idolatry of the nations and became a people who were chosen to serve the one true God. My mother told me that because of them, it was up to me to be different, to be better. For my family, it was not about being religious. It was about being proudly Jewish, about being a good person, about continuing the Jewish people through building a family. An exemplar of Abraham.

In my twenties I finally read the whole book of Genesis. I was disgusted. Certainly, this was not correct! I returned the Bible to my friend Sandra and told her that the Bible was antisemitic because these heroes could not have been such connivers and liars.

Well, Sandra chuckled and said something like, "Andrew, you are them. You are no better than them. That is why I believe these stories are true. Even though God chose them to be the patriarchs, they were still broken people, and God worked through all this brokenness. Abraham was still God's friend. Abraham believed God; God called him righteous. And you can be too even though you are broken like Abraham."

Why didn't anyone tell me this before? I reread the text with fresh eyes and even though I saw murder, deceit, and adultery, I also saw a God of compassion and promise who desires that his people love and serve him and one another. Jews are called to be an example of fidelity to the God of Israel and friends of strangers; friends of the different.

Where does Rafi stand when I consider this ancient and often mysterious text?

One of the most remarkable dynamics in Scripture is found when Abraham asks God, "shall the Judge of the world not do justice?" (Gen 18:25). This is the first time in the Hebrew Bible where we see someone questioning God and his justice: If you are just then you must judge justly. I think about this a lot in relation to Rafi and it is foundational for coming to terms with the Hebrew Bible and difference and disability. "One of the most remarkable features of the Hebrew Bible is not just that people argue with God, but the possibility that people can argue with God and win."[1] This is essential if you want to read the text through a disability lens.

The Hebrew Bible is a narrative told from the standpoint of the different, the poor, the small, the oppressed, the enslaved, the conquered, the defeated. This orientation towards the margins is the subversive genius of the Hebrew Bible, mandating care and compassion for the outsider and the ostracized. This is the core of Israel's vocation as a caring community. "Whoever oppresses the poor shows contempt for their Maker, but whoever is kind to the needy honors God" (Prov 14:31). The poor and needy are synonymous with the disabled. You must care for those who are different from you, because you have been in their place, you were strangers in the land of Egypt (Lev 19:34; Deut 10:19). This is the anchor of disability thinking in the Hebrew Bible.

Why was Israel chosen by God? Not because it was the largest or the strongest but just the opposite: because she was small and weak (Deut 7:7). Israel was chosen to serve God, to "Be holy because I, the Lord your God, am holy" (Lev 19:2). This is the focal point of Israel's vocation and the place where his affection is set. Holiness is the quality that is to guide his people and represents a consistent path to treat each other, animals, the poor, the stranger, and the disabled.

"Do not curse the deaf or put a stumbling block in front of the blind but fear your God. I am the Lord" (Lev 19:14). This foundational law and others for protecting the disabled are absent from other ancient codes, unheard of in other ancient cultures. The value of the disabled person was revolutionary in the Bible, and this is essential to what Israel must include to be a holy people.

---

1. Levenson, *Creation*, 149.

Holiness is how we approach all these issues. It is how we choose, how we make distinctions, and how we draw near to difference and to God. The presence and power of God's call on his people is reflected in a caring community. Their vocation as holy is to care and to receive care.

This is foundational for us as we develop a disability understanding. God is deeply involved, and we can approach him even during the silence of difference and disability.

All our endeavors, passions, and yearnings, the most wicked and most noble, those that give us joy and those that end up in grief, the greatest of blessings and the deepest of pain and disappointment fall into the mysterious depths of God of the Hebrew Bible where there is comfort, but not necessarily comprehension. We as believers experience both sides: an acknowledgement of God's presence and a perception of His silence or absence. Through the Hebrew Bible we meet characters who struggle in the deep end along with the rest of us:

- Rahab, the pagan prostitute who trusted the Lord and was saved.

- Ruth, the immigrant with no inheritance who was redeemed by a distant relative and became part of the royal family.

- Mephibosheth, crippled in both feet, shameful, yet loved on account of someone else and invited to eat at the king's table forever.

- Gomer, the serial adulteress whose husband bought her back from slavery.

- Joshua, the high priest whose filthy garments were replaced with fresh, clean ones.

- Gideon, the insecure warrior.

There is a promise of wisdom if you read it. The text is not static, and it does not behave. The text is alive, breathing, magical, and often a wrestling match with those who love God.

Disability is ubiquitous in the Hebrew Bible, but its meaning, origin, program, and timetable are problematic. You will not find a term that parallels our word "disability." What we find links a dissimilar group of people. The text arranges people in a way that works for society. It does categorize and sometimes exclude (socially, economically, and religiously) based on physical and mental conditions, appearance, vulnerabilities, and particular disease. Disability plays a significant role in the way the Hebrew Bible articulates God's power and holiness and Israel's election. God's power is manifest in the disabled and God's story is there. God uses disability and disability is sometimes transformed in different ways in the Hebrew Bible.

Difference in the Beginning: Genesis

Genesis shakes the ancient world with a bold claim that all humans are made in the image of God. That was and still is revolutionary. In the ancient world to "be made in the image of a god" was a term of exaltation. The Hebrew Bible offers something different and distinct—a radical claim. The implications were stunning to the ancient world: freedom to choose, individual dignity, honor, and worth. Nowhere is the image of God defined explicitly, but it is described in the accounts of creation not so much as what but much more in terms of why. The true distinguishing characteristic of human beings as distinct from other animals is the purpose for which God has created us rather than a quality intrinsic to what we are.

The first purpose is to care. The Lord God took the man and put him in the garden of Eden to work it and take care of it. The second purpose is to take dominion. "God blessed them and said to them, 'Be fruitful and increase in number; fill the earth and subdue it. Rule over the fish in the sea and the birds in the sky and over every living creature that moves on the ground'" (Gen 1:28).

I see this as a parallel mandate to look after each other and the world. To care is to love and to be cared for is to be loved. Care lies in the heart of the human vocation given by God in the Hebrew Bible. This care mirrors God's care over creation and people. This has repercussions for those dependent on others as we are called to receive care and give care. And in this we are to find purpose and satisfaction.

> Let us make man in our image, according to our likeness. They will rule the fish of the sea, the birds of the sky, the livestock, the whole earth, and the creatures that crawl on the earth (1:26). Be fruitful, multiply, fill the earth, and subdue it (1:28). The LORD God took the man and placed him in the garden of Eden to work it and watch over it (2:15).

The first story is that God creates. The second story is that Adam is to tend and keep order (dominion). He is to care for God's good creation. To care is to be human, it is an essential consequence. This is the task God gave to human beings to rule over creation as stewards. Care represents God to the rest of creation. We represent in a tangible, visible way the invisible

God. He is the King over all of creation, and we are his stewards or vice-regents. Our purpose is to be the agents of God's care as it is worked out in his world. Attending to his creatures is attending to God.

There will be periods of injury and diminishment, but the one who receives care has a vocation and the caregiver has a vocation. To have disability or diminishment is not a diminishment of personhood or vocation or dignity. It is a time in life when dominion takes on a form. Any body, and the person occupying it, is still God's and it remains holy and in his image. To be human is to be loved and dependent and to care and be cared for. Caring and being cared for are part of the same command.

There are different ways of being human. This is the filter by which we understand disability. Experiences and differences that we call disability are nothing more or less than the human difference that requires a particular kind of care and love. All bodies are different, and all require different kinds of care and love. If this is true, then inclusion is not just about accessibility. It is about our hearts, knowing that inside there is no difference. Knowing that for God, there is no difference.

When God created Eve, everything was different by necessity. Yet it was only through the presence and closeness of difference that Adam could be saved from his own aloneness. Thanks to God and because of what we see in creation, we are all different and we all belong to one another.

Identifying and Naming

> Now the LORD God had formed out of the ground all the wild animals and all the birds in the sky. He brought them to the man to see what he would name them; and whatever the man called each living creature, that was its name. So, the man gave names to all the livestock, the birds in the sky and all the wild animals. (Gen 2:19–20)

Adam names things by knowing their essence. We have that same responsibility to name things properly. When you reduce or diminish a person by naming only one part of them, it produces alienation and humiliation. Rafi must be named according to what and who he is, not just one part of him. Of course, his difference is profound and significant, but is that all there is about him? He is different compared to what? I'm certain that for all of us, when the time in our lives comes when we can do nothing but be cared for, we will not want to be defined by that. We will want to be named as a person, a mother, a daughter, a sister, with our own characteristics and particularities.

Genesis 2 celebrates the intimacy of companionship, with no reference to sexuality or procreation. It indicates that one of humanity's fundamental needs is to live in relationship with others. People with disabilities of necessity have a profound sense of this truth. Those of us with able bodies maintain an illusion of autonomy, which is inescapably temporary. Limitations, and the vocation of caring and being cared for, serve as a reminder of God's good intent for humans to meet each other's need for friendship and to be one another's helper. Disabilities and a clear awareness of our limitations have the potential to lead us toward greater imagination and connectedness with each other.

Genesis opens with the creation of difference, and in Genesis 11 we can see a challenge to that difference: the effort to impose homogeneity in Babel. Then in Genesis 12 the text shifts again toward difference, when God calls Abraham to be different and his descendants to be set apart for a purpose. How do we understand and cope with these transitions?

Babel serves the text as a turning point. After the builders of Babel tried to impose a sameness on divinely created difference, God decided that Abraham and his descendants were to be different so that difference would be made known and have dignity. The text of the Hebrew Bible is filled with the story of this difference, its humanity and inhumanity, its limitations and its potential.

The Hebrew Bible and Problems with Disability

There are undoubtedly problems, real challenges that confront a disability reader of the text. These problems are not exhaustive: divine agency and rejection, disqualification, stigma, and prophetic utopia. It starts with Moses:

> "I am slow of speech and tongue." The LORD said to him, "Who gave human beings their mouths? Who makes them deaf or mute? Who gives them sight or makes them blind? Is it not I, the LORD? Now go; I will help you speak and will teach you what to say." But Moses said, "Pardon your servant, LORD. Please send someone else." "What about your brother, Aaron the Levite? I know he can speak well. He is already on his way to meet you, and he will be glad to see you. You shall speak to him and put words in his mouth; I will help both of you speak and will teach you what to do.

> He will speak to the people for you, and it will be as if he were your
> mouth and as if you were God to him." (Exod 4:10–16)

Moses is called by God, but he is hesitant to heed the call, admitting to an unidentified speech disability. Moses calls it slow, sluggish, heavy, awkward, thick, or clumsy. Maybe he stammers or stutters. But God seems unimpressed by Moses' reluctance, basically explaining "I made your mouth like this, I will help you." God reminds us that this really isn't about Moses, it's about God. God points the finger at himself in human difference.

While we know little of the lives of those with disability in the Hebrew Bible, the text points us to something essential: divine agency and its relationship to disability.

Divine agency is based in God's perfect attributes and derived from the way God was felt to interact with human beings. In Exodus we saw God understood as having control over speech and hearing and vision: Who gave human beings their mouths? Who makes them deaf or mute? Who gives them sight or makes them blind? Is it not I, the Lord?

Textual Challenges

Disability is clearly considered to be a vulnerability in people that makes them need and deserve protection, as do the poor, the widow, the orphan, and the stranger. As we see in these examples:

> . . . because I rescued the poor who cried for help and the fatherless
> who had none to assist them. The one who was dying blessed me;
> I made the widow's heart sing. I put on righteousness as my clothing; justice was my robe and my turban. I was eyes to the blind and
> feet to the lame. I was a father to the needy; I took up the case of
> the stranger. (Job 29:12–16)

> He upholds the cause of the oppressed and gives food to the hungry. The Lord sets prisoners free, the Lord gives sight to the blind,
> the Lord lifts up those who are bowed down, the Lord loves the
> righteous. The Lord watches over the foreigner and sustains the
> fatherless and the widow, but he frustrates the ways of the wicked.
> (Ps 146:7–9)

Disability comes from God. Disability and sickness are not simply neutral: we have several cases where God inflicts sickness and disability as judgement, as in 1 Samuel 16:14 and 2 Chronicles 26:16–21. It can be a curse that God brings on people who reject his word and refuse to obey him:

> The LORD will afflict you with madness, blindness, and confusion of mind. At midday you will grope about like a blind person in the dark. You will be unsuccessful in everything you do; day after day you will be oppressed and robbed, with no one to rescue you. (Deut 28:28–29)

We read many times in the Hebrew Bible that sacrificial offerings must be of animals without defect. In Deuteronomy this is made explicitly clear: "If an animal has a defect, is lame or blind, or has any serious flaw, you must not sacrifice it to the LORD your God" (Deut 15:21). God seems to want only the physically perfect and rejects the disabled, the imperfect. Even more difficult are the rules for priests in Leviticus 21, where the physically imperfect are forbidden from serving at the altar like other priests:

> Say to Aaron: "For the generations to come none of your descendants who has a defect may come near to offer the food of his God. No man who has any defect may come near: no man who is blind or lame, disfigured or deformed; no man with a crippled foot or hand, or who is a hunchback or a dwarf, or who has any eye defect, or who has festering or running sores or damaged testicles. No descendant of Aaron the priest who has any defect is to come near to present the food offerings to the LORD. He has a defect; he must not come near to offer the food of his God. He may eat the most holy food of his God, as well as the holy food; yet because of his defect, he must not go near the curtain or approach the altar, and so desecrate my sanctuary. I am the LORD, who makes them holy." (Lev 21:18–21)

The text clearly has a strong orientation toward an ideal of physical perfection:

> Then the king ordered [into] the king's service some of the Israelites from the royal family and the nobility, young men without any physical defect, handsome, showing aptitude for every kind of learning, well informed, quick to understand, and qualified to serve in the king's palace. He was to teach them the language and literature of the Babylonians. (Dan 1:3–4)

> You are altogether beautiful, my darling; there is no flaw in you. (Song of Songs 4:7)

Those without defect are beautiful.

Leprosy

Leprosy is a particular case in the Hebrew Bible, a chronic illness that functions like a disability, including humiliation, social isolation, and physical distancing. We meet the leper in a miserable state: clothes torn, head shaven, calling out the words of his disgrace: "Impure! Impure!" And our first instruction is to exile him: "Being impure he shall sit alone; his dwelling shall be outside the camp" (Lev 13:46). The afflicted were quarantined apart from others until it could be determined whether the active and infectious stage of the illness passed. But this state does not last long. Once past, the sufferer could then be declared clean and readmitted to the community. The leper is to be purified through a series of mysterious priestly rituals. He is not cured, but as soon as he undergoes the ritual and bathes, we read: "after that, he shall enter the camp" (Lev 14:8). Precautionary measures are still taken, but he comes back into the camp, among his people. That is the paradigm. That is how the Lord wants us to deal with the leper. Help him. And bring him back in. The mandate is still intact—care.

But some of the ill bear their affliction for life and are permanently excluded from the camp. They are not welcomed back. There must have been persistent mourning as an expression of grief over this isolation. The texts imply that as long as they have the disease, they remain unclean. They must live alone. There must have been a terrible estrangement and alienation from touching and being touched. The leper was one of the four unfortunates considered to suffer a living death.[2]

As if the pain of his isolation were not enough, he is also charged with helping to ensure that the quarantine is not broken. He must proclaim his own impurity so that others are careful not to have any contact. Perhaps this funerary appearance intensified his need to call out while covering part of his face, in order to clarify the nature of his mourning so that others would not approach to comfort. He cries out to enforce his own isolation.

However, some rabbinic interpreters understand the cries in radically different terms. The leper calls out "Impure! Impure!" not to remind others to stay away but to let them "know of his suffering so that they pray for mercy on his behalf" (Babylonian Talmud, Niddah 66a). The sages who offer this interpretation do not feel they can override a biblical mandate to isolate, but they can transform the tone of the separation. The afflicted are cast out but not forgotten. This understanding alters the human dynamic

2. See Babylonian Talmud Nedarim 64b; Sanhedrin 47a; Num 12:12.

between the sick and the rest of the community, seeking to elicit a deeper level of humanity from the community.

This rabbinic reading invites the afflicted not to grant stigma and shame the final word. One who needs divine mercy should ask for it, and one who yearns to know that others care for him should ask for expressions of love and concern. Those who are unafflicted may be tempted to look down on those who are, to see those whose illness is suggestive of death as less than fully human and thus as unworthy of their compassion. The Hebrew Bible reminds them that the ill are no less human. While this text defines the leper as impure, it does not explicitly make a moral judgement on those with leprosy.

Leprosy, like disability, points to our temporariness, our vulnerability, and the eventual corruption of human life. Leprosy, like disability, asks us to consider where we put our hope—do the things of the world matter during this encounter?

Prophetic Utopia

The Hebrew Bible is a complete system for guiding the ancient Israelites in this world, but it is also an image of the future, described particularly in the prophetic books. At the glorious future of God's intervention, we have a vision of an ideal world, in which the disabled are physically transformed by a God who is incomparable in his ability to heal.

> Then will the eyes of the blind be opened and the ears of the deaf unstopped. Then will the lame leap like a deer, and the mute tongue shout for joy. The unclean will not journey on it; wicked fools will not go about on it. Gladness and joy will overtake them, and sorrow and sighing will flee away. (Isa 35:6)

> See, I will bring them from the land of the north and gather them from the ends of the earth. Among them will be the blind and the lame, expectant mothers, and women in labor; a great throng will return. (Jer 31:8)

> I will gather the lame; I will assemble the exiles and those I have brought to grief. I will make the lame my remnant, those driven away a strong nation. The LORD will rule over them in Mount Zion from that day and forever. (Mic 4:6–7)

> At that time, I will deal with all who oppressed you. I will rescue
> the lame; I will gather the exiles. I will give them praise and honor
> in every land where they have suffered shame. (Zeph 3:19)

Thoughts on Job and Disability

Does Job fear God for nothing (Job 1:9)? The implication here is that there is a causal relationship: fearing God brings reward. Job is blessed so he blesses God; if he is cursed, he will curse God and the things of the world are determinative.

Job's body was greatly afflicted when he was being tested, so much so that when his friends saw him from a distance, they could hardly recognize him (Job 2). Job is public—he is visible in his body, and this draws attention to his scars. He does not hide but brings his broken body to God, to his friends and to us. There would have been a universal abhorrence for his physical abnormalities. He would have been shunned. But Job refuses to cover up. He wants everyone to know what has happened. He has nothing to hide. It is his way of being human. "This is who I am." And thus Job draws attention to his disfigurement: "My body is clothed with worms and scabs, my skin is broken and festering. My eyes have grown dim with grief; my whole frame is but a shadow" (Job 7:5; 17:7). He insists that God is answerable. "God has made me a byword to everyone, a man in whose face people spit" (Job 17:6). He is socially alienated: "My breath is offensive to my wife; I am loathsome to my own family" (Job 19:17). But in all this he does not ask to be cured; he asks only for an explanation. How, God, does this fit into your plan?

God eventually meets with Job. God affirms that his condition is worthy of encounter and his fortunes are restored twofold. But nothing is said about bodily restoration. Job's disfigurement is not an aberration to be reversed. It is who he is now. This is his body now. There is an interesting occurrence in Job 42:9, rendered in English that God accepted Job. The Hebrew is more complex: literally that God lifted up Job's face, an image we might hold of God touching the disfigured face of Job.

What we overlook is an uncomplimentary side of Job:

> When I went to the gate of the city and took my seat in the pub-
> lic square, the young men saw me and stepped aside and the old
> men rose to their feet; the chief men refrained from speaking and
> covered their mouths with their hands; the voices of the nobles

were hushed, and their tongues stuck to the roof of their mouths. Whoever heard me spoke well of me, and those who saw me commended me, because I rescued the poor who cried for help, and the fatherless who had none to assist them. The one who was dying blessed me; I made the widow's heart sing. I put on righteousness as my clothing; justice was my robe and my turban. I was eyes to the blind and feet to the lame. I was a father to the needy; I took up the case of the stranger. I broke the fangs of the wicked and snatched the victims from their teeth. I thought, "I will die in my own house, my days as numerous as the grains of sand. My roots will reach to the water, and the dew will lie all night on my branches. My glory will not fade; the bow will be ever new in my hand." (Job 29: 1–20)

But now they mock me, men younger than I, whose fathers I would have disdained to put with my sheep dogs. (Job 30:1)

Job's moral witness is complicated, and it mirrors our own complicated world. He modeled advocacy for the disabled, but he did it for public approval and for exalted status in his community. He has self-indulgent memories of his own importance.

Here we see an ugly and unflattering side of Job. He would not allow his dogs to be with the underclass and he was at the top of his social class. Now he is at the bottom. He wants to help the disabled, but he does not want to be counted among them. He is now incredulous to be one of them. Does his self-importance undermine his testimony? Job's story underlines the fact that intention matters, but the sacredness of the story is not dependent on it. We must consider the cumulative witness of the whole text.

Selected Stories of Disability from the Hebrew Bible

Genesis 27:1

When Isaac was old and his eyes were so weak that he could no longer see, he called for Esau his older son and said to him, "My son . . ."

A simple point is that Isaac's disability did not alter his identity. He was accommodated. He was not powerless or cast aside. He was dependent on care which was received, yet he retained the same authority and his sons responded. Of course, there were ulterior motives, but this is a reminder that we all, ultimately, become disabled in one way or another. The text was not afraid to show it.

Genesis 32:24

> Jacob remained alone. And a man wrestled with him until the break of dawn.

Jacob is fearful and dishonest, a sneak, a usurper. He lies. He steals. He runs. He has material possessions. He is still not really his own person. He lacks legitimacy and integrity. After he prevails in a fight with the stranger and receives his blessing, Jacob becomes disabled when he is injured at the hip. He then received a new name, meaning "he who wrestles with God." That new name reflects struggle, and the destiny of his people. He limps and he is wounded, but victorious. His disability is his name, and he possesses a new integrity. Jacob lives bearing the visible sign of an encounter.

1 Kings 14:4–5

> Now Ahijah could not see; his sight was gone because of his age. But the LORD had told Ahijah, "Jeroboam's wife is coming to ask you about her son, for he is ill, and you are to give her such and such an answer. When she arrives, she will pretend to be someone else."

Ahijah's blindness was not a moral judgment and does not disqualify him from continuing as a prophet with God's endorsement. His disability seems to be integrated into Israel's society and cult. The prophet judges and rebukes Jeroboam's immorality and all that he predicts comes to pass: Jeroboam's sin is the measure of how future kings would be judged.

2 Samuel 4:4; 9:5–13

Jonathan had a son who was lame in both feet. He was five years old when . . . his nurse picked him up; but as she hurried to leave, he fell and became crippled. His name was Mephibosheth . . . When Mephibosheth . . . came before David, he bowed deeply, honoring David. David spoke his name: "Mephibosheth. I'd like to do something special for you in memory of your father Jonathan. I'm returning to you all the properties of your grandfather Saul. From now on you'll take all your meals at my table." Shuffling and stammering, not looking him in the eye, Mephibosheth said, "Who am I that you pay attention to a stray dog like me?" David said, "Everything that belonged to Saul and his family, I've handed over to your master's grandson. You and your sons and your servants will work his land and bring in the produce, provisions for your master's grandson. Mephibosheth himself, your master's grandson, from now on will take all his meals at my table." And Mephibosheth ate at David's table, just like one of the royal family. Mephibosheth also had a small son named Mica. All who were part of Ziba's household were now the servants of Mephibosheth. Mephibosheth lived in Jerusalem, taking all his meals at the king's table. He was lame in both feet.

The story begins with irony. Most kings in the ancient world were admired for an ideal of beauty and strength. Saul's physicality garnered him support for the throne, but his descendent cannot stand on his own. David calls him by name several times. Names are important and there is no reference to his disability until after we are introduced to him. There is no evidence of stigmatization or shame or charity in this encounter. David sends for Mephibosheth, and he is given royal patronage and elevated to a prince. David acts obediently towards God and man. David keeps his promises to Jonathan. He shows mercy. He loves friendship.

Barrenness

Barrenness is the defining female disability in the Hebrew Bible, a condition which afflicted many biblical women, including Sarah, Rebecka, Rachel, Samson's mother, Hannah, and Michal. When Rachel finally conceives after many years of infertility and gives birth to Joseph, she exclaims, "God has taken away my disgrace" (Gen 30:23). Barrenness is presented as something that God is caught up in and responsible for (1 Sam 1:16). Fertility is a blessing, a reward for obedience to God.

Yet as with other disabilities we are invited to envision a future of reversal. Isaiah promises a future glory of Zion, where mourning turns to joy: "Sing, barren woman, you who never bore a child; burst into song, shout for joy, you who were never in labor; because more are the children of the desolate woman than of her who has a husband" (Isa 54:1).

Concluding Thoughts on Disability and Difference in the Hebrew Bible

Despite all the problems of associating disability with shame, stigma, and the marginalized, Judaism's unique conception of ethical monotheism, innovative understanding of covenantal law, and revolutionary messages from the prophets inspire Western civilization's ethical ideals. The texts speak to persistent themes of our times: immigration, the different and the stranger, forgiveness and reconciliation, marriage and sexuality, the environment, the sanctity of life, care for the poor, weak, vulnerable, and disabled, and less privileged, hope for the future despite destruction and exile in this world. Judaism calls it *chesed ve'tzedek*: kindness and justice. These are the cornerstones of Jewish ethics in the Hebrew Bible and the anchors for this foundational understanding of disability:

> Will the judge of all the earth judge rightly? (Gen 18:25)

> For the LORD your God is God of gods and LORD of lords, the great, the mighty, and the awesome God, who is not partial and takes no bribe. He executes justice for the fatherless and the widow, and loves the sojourner, giving him food and clothing. Love the sojourner, therefore, for you were sojourners in the land of Egypt. (Deut 10:17–19)

> He raises up the poor from the dust; he lifts the needy from the ash heap to make them sit with princes and inherit a seat of honor. (1 Sam 2:8)

> He raises the poor from the dust and lifts the needy from the ash heap. (Ps 113:7)

> Speak out for those who cannot speak, for the rights of the destitute. Speak out, judge righteously, defend the rights of the poor and needy. (Prov 31:8–9)

> The LORD, the LORD, a God merciful and gracious, slow to anger, and abounding in steadfast love and faithfulness, keeping steadfast love for thousands, forgiving. (Exod 34:6–7)

> Justice, and only justice, you shall follow, that you may live and inherit the land that the LORD your God is giving you. (Deut 16:20)

> Do not oppress the stranger, the orphan, and the widow. (Deut 24:17, 27:19; Jer 22:3)

What are mere mortals that you should think about them, human beings that you should care for them? Yet you made them only a little lower than God and crowned them with glory and honor. You gave them charge of everything you made, putting all things under their authority. (Ps 8:4–6)

The Scriptures challenge us to a pilgrimage of discovery. When the author of Psalm 8 looked at the immensity and majesty of the cosmos he asked the question "what is mankind that you are mindful of them, human beings that you care for them?" In answering this question, the writer does not attempt to define characteristics of human beings that qualify us to be cared for by God or to care for others. The fact that God cares serves as the model for our care.

Brokenness, the weak, the marginalized, the poor, the disabled: these are at the center. God's reputation is at stake. This is the countercultural message of the Hebrew Bible. God says to Rafi "I am in all of this."

The Lord does not look at the things people look at. People look at the outward appearance, but the Lord looks at the heart. (1 Sam 16:7; 10–11)

Workbook Questions

1. We are often surprised to encounter stories in the Hebrew Bible where people argue with God, calling him to account for our suffering. Think about why this is so often shocking to us. What can this surprise tell us about the ways we have been conditioned to think about and relate to God?

2. Give some examples of how the "dignity of difference" is established in the Hebrew Bible, and its implications for ways of envisioning society.

3. What can the story of Job teach us about ourselves, our relationship to disability, and our relationship with God?

8

Jesus and Difference

> While Jesus was dining at Levi's house, many tax collectors and
> sinners were eating with Him and His disciples—for there were
> many who followed Him. When the scribes who were Pharisees
> saw Jesus eating with these people, they asked His disciples, "Why
> does He eat with tax collectors and sinners?" (Matt 9:10–11; Mark
> 2:15–16; Luke 5:29–30)

A CURSORY READING OF the Gospels will give you an idea of the people
Jesus devotes his time to: fishermen, the sick, a tax collector, the outcast,
a thief, women. Jesus did not seem to resonate with the powerful or the
popular. He enjoys those who were called "sinners." He offers friendship to
people who are different, outsiders. Jesus who lived on the margin was sent
to the marginalized. I imagine he would prefer to be with Rafi rather than
with an important and wealthy person. I wonder if Rafi is the one in the
center and the rest of us are really on the margins.

"Zacchaeus, come down immediately. I must stay at your house today"
(Luke 19:5). What does it mean to eat in someone's house, and especially
the house of a wealthy tax collector, a despised Jewish operative of Rome?
Going into the house of a friend is to give trust and authority to that person.
You become vulnerable. There is an intimacy in being in another person's
home—you have access to their private and privileged place. They have
given this to you. They are giving of their time, exposing themselves and

sacrificing something for their guests. It is the greatest form of proximity to invite a stranger into your home.

Jesus comes to us in disguise and on the periphery. Jesus is the center, yet he comes from the margins and goes to the margins. He was an insignificant, self-taught rabbi from an inconsequential neighborhood in a scorned far corner of a powerful empire that despised the people and the land that they ruled. The Gospels show us outsiders who become insiders, transformed into an inclusive community where Jesus is host.

Jesus challenges us to be in proximity to outliers. By inviting the different to be his friends he invites them into his own home.

Jesus: Healing the Broken

A medicalized worldview is part of our modern Western obsession, offering us an illusion of control over disease and suffering. We imagine we can walk into a hospital with something profoundly wrong, and a waiting doctor who knows exactly what to do will use complex machines and medicines to fix us and send us back out into the world, much like a mechanic who replaces a broken piece with a new one.

Jesus was not a doctor that fixes this and that. He was no mechanic. His healings were compassionate statements about God's redemptive movement through the incarnation. What can we read in Jesus' healings about difference and disability?

Throughout the Gospels Jesus is busy healing the lame and the blind. His interactions with and answers surrounding healing, health, and disability often dismantle assumptions about personal sin and generational impairment, ultimately to emphasize that human difference exists, but is not determinative.

"It is not the healthy who need a doctor but the sick. I have come not to call the righteous but sinners" (Matt 9:12; Mark 2:17; Luke 5:31). The relationship between sin and illness/disability hovers in the background. The religious and social culture of the New Testament believed that difference and disability was a result of sin and moral inferiority, thus something to be avoided and excluded.

Jesus deconstructs this dynamic and replaces it with a new kind of relationship between forgiveness and healing under the authority of Jesus. The active categories are not sin and disability, as a kind of cause and effect.

Rather the dynamic is one of sin and forgiveness, and healing. But forgiveness does not always result in a physical healing, visible to the outside.

This is the true anchor for a theology of difference and disability in the Gospels.

What follows are several examples from different Gospels that can help us to see this dynamic at work.

John: The Man Born Blind

> As he went along, he saw a man blind from birth. His disciples asked him, "Rabbi, who sinned, this man or his parents, that he was born blind?" "Neither this man nor his parents sinned," said Jesus, "but this happened so that the works of God might be displayed in him." (John 9:1–3)

The disciples here stand in for society, asking a question that reflects the prevailing attitude that there was some moral failure at cause. Whether it was the disabled man himself, or his parents, someone must have sinned and brought upon him God's judgment in the form of blindness. This is an assumption grounded in a covenantal understanding that obedience brings blessing and disobedience brings God's curse, and the Torah's understanding of sins of the fathers (Exod 20:5). It is also an assumption that Jesus categorically rejects.

Jesus' emphasis here is not physical disability but on spiritual matters. This physical blindness is contrasted with the moral blindness of the religious leaders. Metaphors of light and darkness are common in the Gospel of John, including:

- The light shines in the darkness, and the darkness has not overcome it. (1:5)

- Whoever follows me will never walk in darkness but will have the light of life. (8:12)

- I am the light of the world. (8:12)

- I have come into the world as a light, so that no one who believes in me should stay in darkness. (12:46)

For John a blind man is a physical metaphor to illustrate those who morally "walk in darkness." It is Jesus who exposes this blindness and brings light. Because of him, the unknowing have sight.

How could a person sin before he was born? In Jewish theology, a person is thought to have been conceived with two inclinations: good and evil struggle for control, and for most people, good wins. But, as this man was blind from his birth, the possibility of some actual sin before birth would be a speculative question. Some sources conjecture that evil might get the upper hand in the womb.[1]

According to the Gospel text, there is no recollection of any man who was born blind having then been healed. And so, it seems to me, what we see in the text is Messianic. The man worships Jesus to acknowledge this: "Lord, I believe," and "he worshiped him." In his confrontation with the Pharisees, themes of sight and blindness, physical and spiritual, come to the fore. These elements allow us to see that there is far more going on than physical disability, but rather blindness is a vehicle for a much larger discourse about sin, moral darkness, and the offer of healing Jesus presents to us all.

Mark: Demons and Community

> They went across the lake to the region of the Gerasenes. When Jesus got out of the boat, a man with an impure spirit came from the tombs to meet him. This man lived in the tombs, and no one could bind him anymore, not even with a chain. For he had often been chained hand and foot, but he tore the chains apart and broke the irons on his feet. No one was strong enough to subdue him. Night and day among the tombs and in the hills, he would cry out and cut himself with stones. When he saw Jesus from a distance, he ran and fell on his knees in front of him. He shouted at the top of his voice, "What do you want with me, Jesus, Son of the Most High God? In God's name don't torture me!" For Jesus had said to him, "Come out of this man, you impure spirit!" Then Jesus asked him, "What is your name? "My name is Legion," he replied, "for we are many." And he begged Jesus again and again not to send them out of the area. A large herd of pigs was feeding on the nearby hillside. The demons begged Jesus, "Send us among the pigs; allow us to go into them." He gave them permission, and the impure spirits came out and went into the pigs. The herd, about two thousand

---

1. See Edersheim, "Life and Times," 177–87. See also Keener, "Cause of Blindness."

in number, rushed down the steep bank into the lake and were drowned. Those tending the pigs ran off and reported this in the town and countryside, and the people went out to see what had happened. When they came to Jesus, they saw the man who had been possessed by the legion of demons, sitting there, dressed and in his right mind; and they were afraid. Those who had seen it told the people what had happened to the demon-possessed man—and told about the pigs as well. Then the people began to plead with Jesus to leave their region. As Jesus was getting into the boat, the man who had been demon-possessed begged to go with him. Jesus did not let him, but said, "Go home to your own people and tell them how much the Lord has done for you, and how he has had mercy on you." So the man went away and began to tell in the Decapolis how much Jesus had done for him. And all the people were amazed. (Mark 5:1–20)

Care for the suffering is a space where the individual and the communal meet. Looking through the lens of disability at the first part of Mark 5 reveals to us some of the challenges and possibilities of this kind of communal care. In this pericope Jesus crosses the lake of Galilee to the region of the Gerasenes, where he encounters a man tormented by demons. Without entering into the question of the objective reality of such supernatural creatures, we can say that in this world the man was functionally disabled and engaging in self-harm, unclothed and howling.

This is the first time Jesus goes into a gentile area. This was a place that was ritually unclean. The men were uncircumcised and pigs were an essential economic resource. Here we meet a man with an unclean spirit. There are three overlapping foci related to mental illness: the man's situation, the community's response, and Jesus' response.

There are several issues to consider: The demons are called legion. A legion is an occupying and military term, a force of some 4,000–6,000 soldiers. Soldiers would often terrorize local communities and villagers would feign madness as a way of protesting. Perhaps the community was frustrated that they lost their indirect form of protest. Perhaps they assumed the demoniac's mental illness was a choice. A predictable opinion would be that he was weak and morally inferior and that he allowed the demons to possess him. People like this were stigmatized, feared, segregated, and sometimes executed.

His community had indeed stepped up and tried to help: the text explains that "no one was strong enough to retrain him" (v. 4). Notwithstanding our discomfort with the notion of restraint, when the man became a danger to himself, the community understood it had a responsibility. He was not just jailed, removed, or executed. His family probably lived in the village. He was taken care of in some way. Someone paid attention. People knew who he was. They recognized him. In some way he was part of the community, albeit on the margins. Because they knew him, they might not have been afraid when they tried to care for him. Despite being socially marginal and isolated, the man remained part of the community. And when the time came that their care was no longer sufficient, it was Jesus who healed him.

It is a bit surprising that following this healing Jesus refuses to allow the grateful man to join him, insisting that he remain with the community and "tell them how much the Lord has done for you, and what mercy he has shown you" (v. 19). We see here again the communal aspect of disability: the man belongs to the community and is an essential piece of its future. Just as they were once responsible for him, now he is responsible to them, to share his deep experience of God's grace with them.

But the healed man will also share something else with the community when he tells of what happened to him: he will communicate his own true identity. In fact, one of the core themes of the Gospel of Mark is that of identity: when is the man Jesus recognized and revealed as the Christ, and by whom? The Gospel is a surprising story of misidentification, where humans—and particularly the humans closest to Jesus—keep getting it wrong.

The problem of identity, and our human tendency to misunderstand others' true natures isn't restricted to the person of Jesus. Mark 5 also shows how we so often tragically misunderstand and misidentify other people, even those close to us. In this story, when viewed through the eyes and words of Jesus, this disabled man is a person (ἀνθρώπου). While undoubtedly a person with a serious problem and limitation, he is a person. But in the eyes of the community, even though they have cared for him for many years, his disability has over time become his identity: he is a "demoniac" (δαιμονισθεὶς).

Once healed, Jesus instructs the man to "go to your own" (πρὸς τοὺς σούς) and in so doing the healed man shares an essential truth about who God is, and who we really are. This man is not a demoniac. He is a person: a person for whom God has shown great love and mercy. We gain new insight if we look at the text medically, socially, and spiritually. It is a story of mental illness and a stigmatized ailment. A story of long-term, consistent care. A story of a compassionate and a confused yet empathetic community. It is a story of healing and a story in which we must honor a personal and community struggle. If we are only able to listen, the disabled can teach us about what it means to be more deeply human, and how God meets all of us—disabled and able-bodied—in the midst of our human struggles and suffering.

Luke: Leprosy and Our Common Future

> While Jesus was in one of the towns, a man came along who was covered with leprosy. When he saw Jesus, he fell with his face to the ground and begged him, "Lord, if you are willing, you can make me clean." Jesus reached out his hand and touched the man. "I am willing," he said. "Be clean!" And immediately the leprosy left him. Then Jesus ordered him, "Don't tell anyone, but go, show yourself to the priest and offer the sacrifices that Moses commanded for your cleansing, as a testimony to them." Yet the news about him spread all the more, so that crowds of people came to hear him and to be healed of their sicknesses. But Jesus often withdrew to lonely places and prayed. (Luke 5:12–16)
>
> Now on his way to Jerusalem, Jesus traveled along the border between Samaria and Galilee. As he was going into a village, ten men who had leprosy met him. They stood at a distance and called out in a loud voice, "Jesus, Master, have pity on us!" When he saw them, he said, "Go, show yourselves to the priests." And as they went, they were cleansed. One of them, when he saw he was healed, came back, praising God in a loud voice. He threw himself at Jesus' feet and thanked him—and he was a Samaritan. (Luke 17:11–16)

As a chronic condition, leprosy carried with it a sense of hopelessness. But the rituals of Leviticus that Jesus points to in both texts implied the possibility of a cure or at least a dormant phase. Leprosy, like most disability, was traced to a moral cause and the agency of God, regarded as a sign of divine judgment. Lepers entered the synagogue first and left last. Jewish symbolism saw in the sufferings of Israel and the destruction of the temple the fulfillment of the punishment of leprosy.

As we saw earlier, lepers were the ultimate outsiders in ancient Israel, forced into social distancing. The ancient world assumed the condition was contagious. The person with leprosy had to tear his clothing and warn people as he approached: "Unclean . . . unclean!" Those suffering from this illness were temporarily ostracized from society and required to keep their faces covered. They could not enter the temple, and they could not be touched.

When we see Luke 5:12 "a man full of leprosy," we understand a man who has suffered with this for a long time. Jesus touches the man. He rejects the social boundary. It was probably the first time the man was touched since he was declared a leper.

The purification process that Jesus was referring to in these texts are found in Leviticus 13 and 14. Only a priest who was properly trained could verify the man's condition. After his healing Jesus urges him to tell no man but tell the leaders. Jesus wanted the leaders to take him seriously and to confirm his Messianic authority.

Leprosy was a form of living death. It reminds me of the Gregorian chant, written in 1300: "In the midst of life we are in death."[2] We will all suffer the same fate: "All flesh is like grass, and all its glory like the flowers of the field; the grass withers and the flowers fall" (Isa 40:6). We all wear out, become corrupted, and we are all mortal. In a figurative way, leprosy gives us all a glimpse of the future, reminding us that, in Radner's words, it is a disease "in which we are involved and that describes us."[3]

In Jesus' confrontations with leprosy, we receive confidence that he will eventually halt corruption and disintegration. The promise is that corruption of the flesh will end:

> Go back and report to John what you hear and see: The blind receive sight, the lame walk, those who have leprosy are cleansed, the deaf hear, the dead are raised, and the good news is proclaimed to the poor. (Matt 11:4–5)

Into this world of physical, social, and moral corruption Jesus approaches and makes himself known. He eventually offers his own body for it. Those with bodies that are different or disabled, those who are weak or poor, those who are struggling with sin—all can take comfort. Jesus comes to confront and overcome the corruption of Job's flesh.[4] The final hope of Job is 19:26: "And after my skin has been destroyed, yet in my flesh I will see God."

Radner calls this hope the "promise embedded in the disease."[5] The paradox is that God makes us and will heal us. With the coming of the

---

2. White, *Notes and Queries*, 177–78.
3. Radner, *Leviticus*, 136.
4. Radner, *Leviticus*, 144.
5. Radner, *Leviticus*, 144.

Messiah Jesus, "cleanness is directive; it moves by and towards this promise and reality of God's creative intention and nature."[6] Leprosy, diseases of all kinds, and Down syndrome provide a hint of something that is to follow for all of humanity: that all will be gathered together and taken into the body of the Messiah, healed and whole.

Luke-Acts: Inviting the Different

The Gospel of Luke specifically highlights difference. The author seems eager to emphasize narratives about people who don't belong: Samaritans, gentiles, women, the poor, disabled, and vulnerable, tax collectors and sinners. To do so, Luke makes use of pairings that serve to gently throw us off balance and upend convention: male and female, Jews and gentiles, religious and unbelieving, rich and poor, clean and unclean. In mobilizing these pairings, Luke liberates, subverts, and topples our expectations.

Luke shows Jesus encountering those who are perceived to be morally inferior and culturally excluded: the lame and the blind. This is the ultimate power and appeal of Luke's Gospel. It is a reversal of expectancy. Those who share in the kingdom of God are not what one would expect. But this surprise focus is precisely in keeping with Luke's universal message of salvation to all, regardless of ability or difference.

The centurion of Luke 7 highlights a reverse of expectancy. Notice the pairs in this section: The elders and the centurion. Jesus and the elders. Jews and gentiles. The disciples and the people. The crowds and the disciples and the authorities.

The other significant pairing is to be found the location. Capernaum is a place of darkness and unbelief, chosen by Luke as the place to display the centurion's faith. Why would the elders of the Jews go to a rabbi they did not trust on behalf of a man they despised? A man who they assumed was on the margins even though he was powerful?

The centurion had built the synagogue, yet he could not enter the synagogue. He was uncircumcised and unclean, but the elders said he was deserving. Convention is reversed and turned upside down.

We find a similar reversal of expectation in another pericope, later in Luke 7:

6. Radner, *Leviticus*, 145.

One of the Pharisees asked Jesus to eat with him, and he went into the Pharisee's house and took his place at the table. And a woman in the city, who was a sinner, having learned that he was eating in the Pharisee's house, brought an alabaster jar of ointment. She stood behind him at his feet, weeping, and began to bathe his feet with her tears and to dry them with her hair. Then she continued kissing his feet and anointing them with the ointment. Now when the Pharisee who had invited him saw it, he said to himself, "If this man were a prophet, he would have known who and what kind of woman this is who is touching him—that she is a sinner." (Luke 7:36–39)

This raises some acute questions for the reader. Why would a Pharisee ask Jesus to eat with him? The offer of hospitality is radical. Jesus is inside, yet outside. Who was this woman and why was she invited to the home? Was she a prostitute? She is inside, yet outside. Was she already in the home? For the woman to sit at Jesus' feet—and for him to allow her to do so—was controversial. She took the place of a disciple, sitting at the feet of the teacher.

We are equally surprised by the story of the Ethiopian eunuch in Acts 8. Here was a man who was literate, educated, wealthy, black, religious, and castrated. Luke, again, is looking to upend convention. He is interested in the whole person, not just categories.

Now an angel of the Lord said to Philip, "Go south to the road— the desert road—that goes down from Jerusalem to Gaza." So he started out, and on his way he met an Ethiopian eunuch, an important official in charge of all the treasury of the Kandake (which means "queen of the Ethiopians"). This man had gone to Jerusalem to worship, and on his way home was sitting in his chariot reading the Book of Isaiah the prophet. The Spirit told Philip, "Go to that chariot and stay near it." Then Philip ran up to the chariot and heard the man reading Isaiah the prophet. "Do you understand what you are reading?" Philip asked. "How can I," he said, "unless someone explains it to me?" So he invited Philip to come up and sit with him. This is the passage of Scripture the eunuch was reading: "He was led like a sheep to the slaughter, and as a lamb before its shearer is silent, so he did not open his mouth. In his humiliation he was deprived of justice. Who can speak of his descendants? For his life was taken from the earth." The eunuch asked Philip, "Tell me, please, who is the prophet talking about, himself or someone else?" Then Philip began with that very passage of Scripture and told him the good news about Jesus. As they traveled along the road, they came to some water and the eunuch said, "Look, here is water. What can stand in the way of my being baptized?" And he gave orders to stop the chariot. Then both Philip and the eunuch went down into the water and Philip baptized him. When they came up out of the water, the Spirit of the Lord suddenly took Philip away, and the eunuch did not see him again, but went on his way rejoicing. (Acts 8:26–39)

The combination of "eunuch" together with the title "court official" indicates a literal eunuch, who might have been excluded from the temple by the restriction in Deuteronomy 23:1. No one who has been emasculated by crushing or cutting may enter the assembly of the Lord.

Yet there is a hope associated with his disability. This man loved the God of Israel and his word: he was reading and toiling through the prophet Isaiah. He went on his way rejoicing. He might have been seen as an outsider and unclean, but he became an insider who was clean. He might have thought himself unworthy, but he was worthy. He might have been excluded, but he was included. He was not on the margins; he was at home.

Finally, in the story of the woman bent over (Luke 13:10–17) and that of Zacchaeus (Luke 19:1–10) we have encounters with Jesus that undermine and reverse conventions about physical stature. Jesus destabilizes all expectancy. These two people would have likely been judged by their body in relation to size or stature; the woman "bent over" and the man "short." These two would have been assessed in character or personality solely from their outer appearance. Both experience reversals.

The woman was bent, and she is now straight. Her physical stature is restored, and she is healed. She praises God and goes home for the Sabbath. She is called a daughter of Abraham while synagogue leaders are shamed. Notice the contrasting pairs: poor and rich, woman and man, bent and straight, shame and delight.

Zacchaeus experiences reversal from wealthy to almsgiver. His body is the same. He is not healed but now he is included. He was an outsider but now he is inside. Zacchaeus went from being morally suspect, religiously and socially alienated, to being called a son of Abraham and a friend of Jesus. Jesus calls them both by their true names—son or daughter of Abraham—and not according to their appearance.

Jesus preaches "the good news to the poor, to release the oppressed, and to proclaim the year of the Lord's favor" (Luke 4:18–19). The gospel message is good news for all, but especially for the poor, the crippled, the blind, and the lame. There is no barrier of human difference. The outcasts of society wholeheartedly accept Jesus' message. The poor, the crippled, the lame, and the blind are unexpected disciples and welcomed participants in the kingdom.

Luke: Different Ways of Knowing

For Luke, difference is central to our social condition. In keeping with this foundation, Luke-Acts does not privilege one sense, but rather presents multiple valid ways of knowing. This is especially important for a theology of disability. We live in a world that is hyper-conceptual, where a particular type of learning and a specific kind of intelligence is valued, a situation that excludes people like Rafi. Rafi cannot enter a classroom and take notes, do research, and write papers. He cannot participate in the same way that others might be able to. But the fact that he cannot learn in this particular way does not mean he cannot learn and know. He learns and knows differently.

We can see examples of where Luke asserts multiple, complementary ways of knowing. In his telling of the story of healing the blind beggar, the Gospel gives us a different perspective than the account of healing Bartimaeus in Mark's Gospel:

> As Jesus approached Jericho, a blind man was sitting by the roadside begging. When he heard the crowd going by, he asked what was happening. They told him, "Jesus of Nazareth is passing by." He called out, "Jesus, Son of David, have mercy on me!" Those who led the way rebuked him and told him to be quiet, but he shouted more, "Son of David, have mercy on me!" Jesus stopped and ordered the man to be brought to him. When he came near, Jesus asked him, "What do you want me to do for you? "Lord, I want to see," he replied. Jesus said to him, "Receive your sight; your faith has healed you." Immediately he received his sight and followed Jesus, praising God. When all the people saw it, they also praised God. (Luke 18: 35–43)

Luke is interested in the body, and there is a great deal of somatic action taking place: approaching, sitting, begging, hearing, going, calling, asking, wanting, bringing, persisting, shouting, replying, following, glorifying. For Luke nothing is privileged in encountering and witnessing the work of the Spirit.

The same is true of Luke's account on the road to Emmaus:

Now that same day two of them were going to a village called Emmaus, about seven miles from Jerusalem. They were talking with
each other about everything that had happened. As they talked
and discussed these things with each other, Jesus himself came up
and walked along with them; but they were kept from recognizing
him. He asked them, "What are you discussing together as you
walk along?" They stood still, their faces downcast. One of them,
named Cleopas, asked him, "Are you the only one visiting Jerusalem who does not know the things that have happened there in
these days?" "What things?" he asked. "About Jesus of Nazareth,"
they replied. "He was a prophet, powerful in word and deed before
God and all the people. The chief priests and our rulers handed
him over to be sentenced to death, and they crucified him; but we
had hoped that he was the one who was going to redeem Israel.
And what is more, it is the third day since all this took place. In
addition, some of our women amazed us. They went to the tomb
early this morning but didn't find his body. They came and told us
that they had seen a vision of angels, who said he was alive. Then
some of our companions went to the tomb and found it just as
the women had said, but they did not see Jesus." He said to them,
"How foolish you are, and how slow to believe all that the prophets have spoken! Did not the Messiah have to suffer these things
and then enter his glory?" And beginning with Moses and all the
Prophets, he explained to them what was said in all the Scriptures
concerning himself. As they approached the village to which they
were going, Jesus continued on as if he were going farther. But
they urged him strongly: "Stay with us, for it is nearly evening; the
day is almost over." So he went in to stay with them. When he was
at the table with them, he took bread, gave thanks, broke it and
began to give it to them. Then their eyes were opened and they
recognized him, and he disappeared from their sight. They asked
each other, "Were not our hearts burning within us while he talked
with us on the road and opened the Scriptures to us?" They got up
and returned at once to Jerusalem. There they found the Eleven
and those with them, assembled together and saying, "It is true!
The Lord has risen and has appeared to Simon." Then the two told
what had happened on the way, and how Jesus was recognized by
them when he broke the bread. (Luke 24:13–35)

Again, the text is extremely bodily: the two of them were walking,
going, talking, discussing. Jesus is asking and they stood waiting. They were
downcast and he explained. They heard and saw. They approached, were
going, and urging. They stayed, they went, they saw, they ate, then their

eyes opened. Jesus disappeared. There hearts were burning. They got up and they returned. This text shows all these characteristics: seeing, standing, hearing, hearts, looking, touching, hoping, amazing, finding, telling, vision, going, suffering, entering, explaining, saying, urging, staying, eating, giving, opening, recognizing. Nothing is particularly privileged in communication or understanding. There are many ways.

Finally, we see this multisensory modality at its most active at Pentecost.

> When they heard this sound, a crowd came together in bewilderment, because each one heard their own language being spoken . . . "We hear them declaring the wonders of God in our own tongues!" (Acts 2:6; 11)

Again, we see a strong somatic interest: people sitting and resting, speaking in other tongues, hearing this sound, being bewildered in their hearing, feeling amazed and perplexed. The text continues:

> In the last days, God says, I will pour out my Spirit on all people. Your sons and daughters will prophesy, your young men will see visions, your old men will dream dreams. Even on my servants, both men and women, I will pour out my Spirit in those days, and they will prophesy. I will show wonders in the heavens above and signs on the earth below, blood and fire and billows of smoke. The sun will be turned to darkness and the moon to blood before the coming of the great and glorious day of the Lord. And everyone who calls on the name of the Lord will be saved. (Acts 2:17–21, quoting from Joel 2:28–32)

We notice many things happening here: people seeing, hearing, dreaming, showing, wonders, signs, sun, moon, blood, fire, darkness, and calling. Information is received through a multiplicity of diverse phenomena, actions, and senses. Pentecost is not limited to speech or hearing. There are many tongues and many senses used. All of these modes should be conduits for communication. Vision is precisely the intersection of language, ability, and disability.

Pentecost shows us the many ways that the spirit works and speaks, in different ways, and to everyone. All people truly means everyone—no one is missed or forgotten. Discipleship must be patient about what people will become versus what they are now. We must see the specific, individual person in front of us. Pentecost insists on this. And on the need to wait. Unfortunately we in churches today emphasize creed, belief, and commitments to intellectual positions and propositional truths. The more this is the focus, the more the disabled are marginalized. Let us keep an eye on Pentecost, where everyone has a place and everyone has a way to experience and communicate the Spirit.

Matthew and Luke: The Great Feast

> I say to you that many will come from the east and the west and will take their places at the feast with Abraham, Isaac and Jacob in the kingdom of heaven. But the subjects of the kingdom will be thrown outside, into the darkness, where there will be weeping and gnashing of teeth. (Matt 8:11–12)

Perhaps the prevailing belief was that at the end of the age, there would be a big feast welcoming the Messiah, and that the patriarchs would be the hosts. The assumption would be that the Jewish people—the physical children of Abraham—would have their tickets stamped and paid for this feast. Yet Jesus says that many will come from the east and west.

Who is invited to the banquet? Everyone. Who is excluded from the banquet? Surprisingly, the children of Abraham. They are excluded because Jesus is turning convention on its head. The price for the ticket is not birthright. You get a ticket because you are his friend.

Then Jesus said to his host,

> When you give a luncheon or dinner, do not invite your friends, your brothers or relatives, or rich neighbors; if you do, they may invite you back and so you will be repaid. But when you give a banquet, invite the poor, the crippled, the lame, the blind, and you will be blessed. Although they cannot repay you, you will be repaid at the resurrection of the righteous. (Luke 14:12–14)

The parable of the great banquets' call is to "Go out at once into the streets and lanes of the town and bring in the poor, the crippled, the blind, and the lame" (Luke 14:21). People with impairments of all kinds are not invisible or erased. They still carry the marks of their difference. Blemished and non-blemished, all are welcome. The disabled are honored: their particular features of brokenness are not eliminated or eradicated but redeemed.

People who are different and with disabilities have a vital role in the kingdom. Christ points to them as examples of humility and genuine discipleship. The mandate to care for the outcast is part of the call to be a disciple. The parable has less to do with the disabled and more to do with the religious and social hierarchy that perpetuated discrimination against the poor and the disabled. Jesus closed his comments with the reminder that the poor might not be able to repay their hosts, but the hosts would be repaid at the resurrection.

When one of those at the table with him heard this, he said to Jesus, "Blessed is the man who will eat at the feast in the kingdom of God" (Luke 14:15).

The implication at the close of this parable was that some of these leaders themselves would not even make the guest list: "I tell you, not one of those men who were invited will get a taste of my banquet" (Luke 14:24). The Lord's message was and is striking, convicting, and foreboding.

That message is for we who exclude the disabled. We who are normal always have the power over definitions and classifications. The disabled often must accept our definition. Rafi accepts whatever definition is given. The problem is not giving him the chance to define things for himself. The problem is in giving authority to convention, not to the person in front of us. The dominant group seeks to preserve authority. Is this real inclusion and belonging or just charity? How do they become us? By Jesus' invitation of the marginal to his table, the dominant group becomes vulnerable and codependent. Those on the margins become the core and those at the core are moved to the margins. The place where Jesus goes and is invited is the new core.

The Cross and Difference

The image of our religious conviction is the cross—Jesus' body hanging on the cross, where the king of glory suffered and was broken. Our primary image is not one of an able-bodied God: we face a broken and disabled body, and we assert that in this broken body there is a message of grace.

The choice of this symbol as a reminder is startling. It was regarded with horror and shame in the ancient world, the memory of the crucified damned to oblivion. Yet it took hold immediately as the central symbol of our faith, such that around the year 200 CE Tertullian could write of its popularity, such that,

> At every step forward and movement, at every going in and out,
> when we put on our clothes and shoes, when we bathe, when we

> sit at table, when we light the lamps, on couch, on seat, in all the ordinary actions of daily life, we trace upon the forehead, the sign of the cross.[7]

Jesus links his suffering on the cross to the plan of God. Speaking with two followers on the road to Emmaus, he said, "Did not the Messiah have to suffer these things and then enter his glory? And beginning with Moses and all the Prophets, he explained to them what was said in all the Scriptures concerning himself" (Luke 24:26–27).

Paul boasts in the cross in Galatians 6:14, "May I never boast except in the cross of our Lord Jesus Christ, through which the world has been crucified to me, and I to the world." In Jesus' body on the cross there is life in death, through rebirth and transformation.

Today things are different. We live in a time when power is praised, and weakness is derided. The world ridicules the claim that God's anointed suffered on a cross.

Jesus' body was the same as ours in every way. He identifies with us and is aware of the uncertainty and the precarious nature of human life. Yet his body was also different: he could not be broken for us if his body were just like ours. This theological model serves to remind us that the body which is most important is that of Jesus. His body was like and unlike ours, and through reflection on his body we begin to understand our own bodies with all their differences.

"This is my body broken for you" is a picture of a gift of grace through a broken body. He identifies with every aspect of our brokenness. He chose not only brokenness in that he became flesh in life but also that the resurrected Christ still bears the bodily marks of the cross. The affirmation of Jesus' body is an affirmation that those with different, broken bodies still participate in the image of God, confirming nonconventional bodies as whole.[8] He who was physically tortured arose from the dead, and is present in heaven and on earth, at once disabled and whole. His wounds are visible and so we should not be ashamed that ours are as well.

When we recite his words, "Do this in remembrance of me," we remember the broken God who is present. The radically inclusive meaning of the Eucharist must be realized. Anthony Stiff explores the value of John Calvin's eucharistic theology and applies it to the participation of someone like Rafi. For Calvin, communion with God takes place through

7. Marucchi, "Archaeology of the Cross."

8. Eiesland, *Disabled God*, 87.

participation in the eucharistic meal. This is the very substance of the church's fellowship. What takes place in the eucharistic meal is that Jesus shares his presence with his children.

The Eucharist is participation in Christ's broken body. It reminds all disciples that he is the goal and the way of their journey: we do not just remember his body; we are present with his body. Our attention is drawn to the body that defines all bodies.[9] Communion "eclipses all horizontal socializations and stigmatizations that are based upon human power, independence, and perfections."[10] The Eucharist belongs to everyone who has been adopted in Christ. It serves to remind Rafi and us all that the most important body is that of Christ.

As we think about Jesus' body broken for us, we begin to understand our own bodies, which are so different yet so completely the same—so human and so mortal. For Calvin, the inclusion that is most important is the one encountered as we partake in the Eucharist.[11] We are a people who are called to delight in our weaknesses and vulnerabilities. Rafi can and should participate and feel part of this community.

The Incarnation and the Trinity, and the Disabled

> The LORD appeared to Abraham near the large trees of Mamre. Abraham was sitting at the entrance to his tent. It was the hottest time of the day. Abraham looked up and saw three men standing nearby . . . (Gen 18:1–2)

The *Visitation of Abraham and Sarah* is one of the most popular icons in Eastern Christianity. It is said to represent the Trinity: a picture of unity, harmony, interrelation, and invitation.

9. Stiff, "Abiding Value," 143.

10. Stiff, "Abiding Value," 143.

11. Stiff, "Abiding Value," 143.

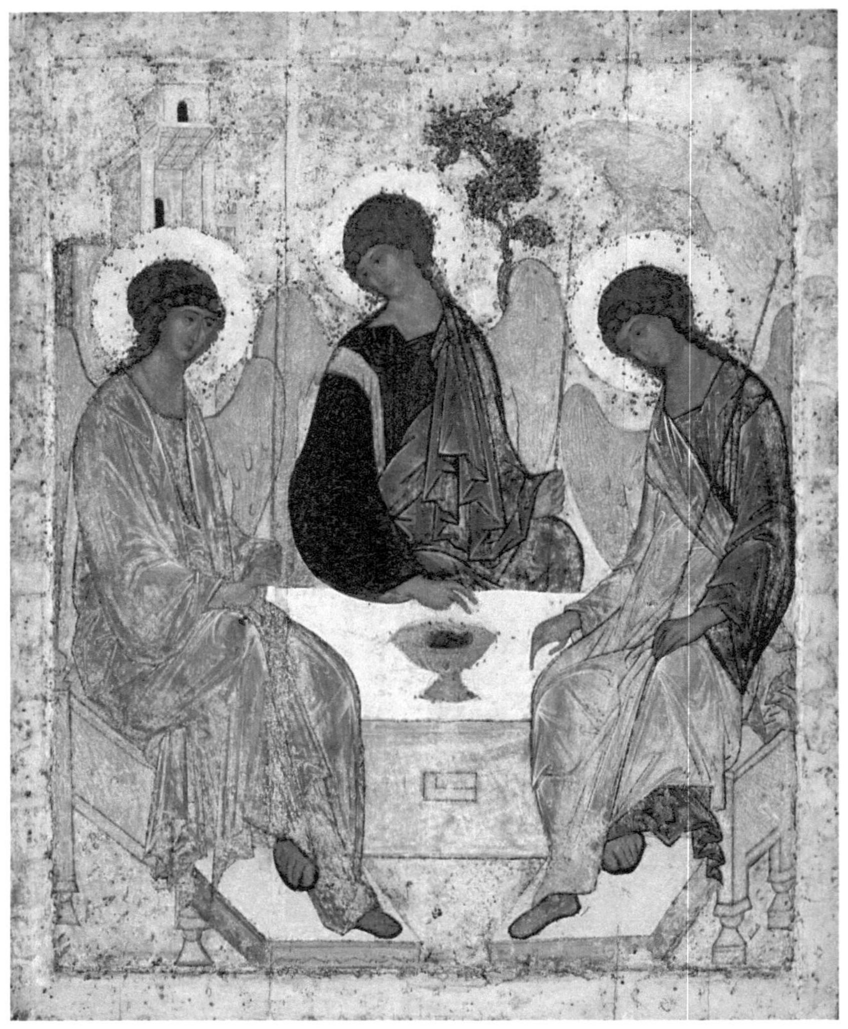

Visitation of Abraham and Sarah

The New Testament develops this in Philippians 2:5–11:

> Who, being in very nature God, did not consider equality with
> God something to be used to his own advantage; rather, he made
> himself nothing by taking the very nature of a servant, being made
> in human likeness. And being found in appearance as a man, he
> humbled himself by becoming obedient to death—even death on

a cross! Therefore God exalted him to the highest place and gave him the name that is above every name, that at the name of Jesus every knee should bow, in heaven and on earth and under the earth, and every tongue acknowledge that Jesus Christ is Lord, to the glory of God the Father.

God is said to be "three-personal," one essence (God) subsisting in three Persons. The Trinity is itself an icon of hospitality, and a celebration of embracing difference.[12] We know that God is love and we are invited to participate in this community of love, and of the *shalom* that is peace and wholeness. God is a community of persons engaged in the eternal, dynamic exchange of love. As Christians, our single most important mission in life is to enter into this intimate pattern of exchange ourselves.

Maximus the Confessor writes of this intimacy: "The union of humanity and divinity . . . does not transform or dissolve God into man or man into God; this conquest is called love."[13] Maximus contends that the ambition of human life is to model the Trinity—to model love. This is a love only desiring the benefit of the beloved. This is love at the core of our life as lived in time. We are not just waiting for death—we are called to love, and to love like God does, because he sent the Son. It cost him everything yet benefitted him nothing. It cost us nothing yet benefitted us everything.

That is the model that inspires me as I love Rafi. There is not much that Rafi can give me besides himself. I only desire his benefit and don't look for anything out of it except his presence in my life.

When disability is manifested in oppositional terms between those who are able and powerful and those who are disabled and powerless, the result is sin. My care for Rafi is not a charitable activity. Correctly understood I am giving compassionate care for an equal. This is simply my interaction with another person made in the image of God. Our challenge is to come to an understanding of disability in a way that reflects the mystery of the relationships inside Trinity: difference, unity, and love. This is what we should aspire to as we seek proximity to difference and disability.

12. Tataryn and Truchan-Tataryn, *Discovering Trinity in Disability*, 123.

13. Tataryn and Truchan-Tataryn, *Discovering Trinity in Disability*, 63.

Concluding Thoughts on Jesus and Difference

[H]e showed them his hands and side. The disciples were overjoyed when they saw the Lord. So the other disciples told him, "We have seen the Lord!" But he said to them, "Unless I see the nail marks in his hands and put my finger where the nails were, and put my hand into his side, I will not believe." A week later his disciples were in the house again, and Thomas was with them. Though the doors were locked, Jesus came, and he said to Thomas, "Put your finger here; see my hands. Reach out your hand and put it into my side. Stop doubting and believe." (John 20:20–27)

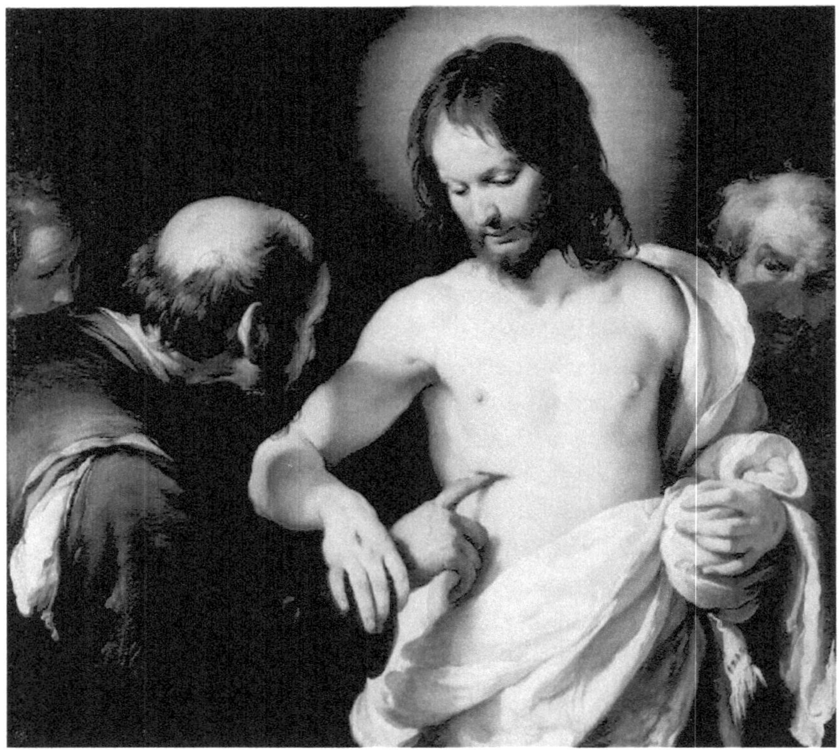

The Incredulity of Saint Thomas

In *The Incredulity of Saint Thomas*, Thomas's posture shows astonishment while Jesus opens his cloak and calmly guides his finger into his wounded side. This is our model. We are Thomas, approaching the vulnerability and wounds of others. And we too can learn to offer our wounds to a scarred and scared world for the healing of others—and ultimately ourselves. The risen Messiah still carries the wounds of the resurrection. He brings his disability with him. The redeemed body is both perishable and imperishable at the same time. Disability does not contradict the human-divine integrity, it becomes a new model of wholeness and a symbol of solidarity.

When Christ came into the world, he said: "Sacrifice and offering you did not desire, but a body you prepared for me" (Heb 10:5). This is who God is. The body is not a worthless container. God gives us of himself as a human with a physical body, and then gives his broken body away for us. His broken body is not an obstacle, but a manifestation of that wholeness.

There is continuity between Jesus' incarnate body and his resurrected body, and we find the same continuity between our present body with its scars and experiences, and the future. The continuity of Jesus' marked body is what confirms his identity. They are tragic and glorious marks, and it is these marks which give us hope, the preservation of our wounds and scars, and the marks of encounters that have characterized our limited existence.

It's hard to imagine the nature of our own resurrected bodies. Will Rafi's resurrected body still bear the marks of Down syndrome? If not, how will I recognize him?

Knowing their thoughts, Jesus said,

> Why do you entertain evil thoughts in your hearts? Which is easier: to say, "Your sins are forgiven," or to say, "Get up and walk"? But I want you to know that the Son of Man has authority on earth to forgive sins. So he said to the paralyzed man, "Get up, take your mat and go home." (Matt 9:4–7)

The peace of God is something much greater than physical healing. While a medicalized worldview sees Jesus as a doctor who fixes broken people, the faithful see healing as an authentication of God's redemption in the incarnation. Scripture reminds us that in Jesus lies true *shalom*: He is the "prince of peace" (Isa 9:6) and "He Himself is our peace" (Eph 2:14). Believers assert that in Messiah there is harmony, wholeness, completeness, prosperity, welfare, and tranquility.

Rafi is healthy, but at the same time he is not. His body is well, but his mind is not. He has anxiety and he is unable to properly regulate his emotions. He is obsessive and compulsive, is easily enraged. Rafi is mercurial. We have been on a long journey of therapy and medicine. There is indeed *shalom*, but not fully. Not yet.

Rafi's body is different. He was made that way and it should be celebrated as such. The Gospels are a testament to the celebration of different bodies and how Jesus interacts with them. Jesus' model of health was not an absence of disability. It is not the absence of disease or suffering. It is the presence of God. Healing is about connecting and reconnecting people to God and their community.

Workbook Questions

1. How might Jesus' healings of the blind and lame be a potential source of misunderstanding in terms of thinking about disability?

2. What can "healing" mean? Are there ways to understand "healing" that are better (or worse) for thinking about disability?

3. What can some of the examples of illness and healing in the New Testament tell us about community and our relationship and responsibility to the disabled?

9

Paul and Difference

His words caused riots and many thought him irrational, deluded, mad, foolish, and frenzied. When he spoke in public he sometimes would be tossed out, lashed, and stoned. His letters resulted in angry exchanges and disputes. His communications were inadequately edited, disjointed and often opaque. Sometimes he changes subjects in the middle of sentences and uses unclear and unexplained metaphors. Paul was brilliant, strident, passionate. He also seems to have sometimes been in a muddle, disorganized and confused even about his own motives and actions. He was misunderstood. He obviously had problems with scheduling. He was frequently distracted and had other problems like shipwrecks, getting arrested, changing direction at the behest of visions and other unplanned interruptions. He was impetuous, impulsive, and unconventional. He claimed to hear God speaking. He had visionary experiences and manifested spiritual gifts such as healings, casting out demons, and confrontations with false prophets.

Despite all this, he helped to organize many churches throughout the Roman Empire. His writings have been translated into over 1,500 languages. Some would say his books are the most dominant in all of literature.

This was Saul of Tarsus—the apostle Paul. He lived with no small number of internal and external challenges. He was almost certainly disabled in some way. And he made that disability the cornerstone of his awareness that weakness and infirmity were foundational to the work of Jesus on the cross.

Power and Weakness

Paul had a counterintuitive theory of power in weakness: Jesus on the cross was powerful, yet weak. In response to the question of are we (Jews) better than them (gentiles), Paul quite simply asserts that we all have the same challenge and we are all judged equally, regardless of our background. "What shall we conclude, then? Do we have any advantage? Not at all! For we have already made the charge that Jews and Gentiles alike are all under the power of sin" (Rom 3:9).

Whatever sense of superiority a reader might have, is put to rest. Any thought of advantage or privilege through Abraham is corrected. God judges justly all people, regardless of their ability, intellect, inheritance, or difference.

In Paul's world, not unlike our own, people met the demands of life by mastering, competing, and seeking advantage. We distinguish ourselves and others between the weak and the strong. Some, like women and slaves, the poor, the disabled, the sick, the stranger, were thought to be weak by definition. But shockingly it is not only that heritage doesn't matter to God—we see here that God specifically chooses and makes use of the lowly, the despised, the weak, and the foolish.

> God chose the foolish things of the world to shame the wise; God chose the weak things of the world to shame the strong. God chose the lowly things of this world and the despised things—and the things that are not—to nullify the things that are. (1 Cor 1:27–27)

God has turned prevailing physical, economic, political, and religious assumptions on their head. When Paul asserts that "there is no longer slave or free, male, or female" (Gal 3:28), he was envisioning a radically countercultural construction of equality gathered around the crucified and anointed one.

Paul enjoins us to enter into solidarity with this difference: we are heirs of God and co-heirs with Christ, if indeed we share in his sufferings in order that we may also share in his glory (Rom 8:17). We enter this community giving preference and honor to the weak.

God acknowledges and receives to himself his physically maimed and socially outcast Son. We see that strength, power, and standing are not conditions of our relationship with God. On the contrary, they can serve as barriers. The marginal, the weak, the intellectually different and the disabled experience God's love and mercy just as does everyone, and Paul's hypocognitive understanding offers the possibility of a language for the wordless:

In the same way, the Spirit helps us in our weakness. We do not know what we ought to pray for, but the Spirit intercedes for us through wordless groans. And he who searches our hearts knows the mind of the Spirit, because the Spirit intercedes for God's people in accordance with the will of God (Rom 8:26). Groanings are not comprehensible speech. But they are not random or meaningless speech, even if wordless. Groanings have "content meaning and intent . . . they . . . transcend articulated formulation."[1]

Rafi cannot recite or deliver the creeds. He cannot assent clearly to any dogma or doctrine. His expressive language is often rambling and incoherent to us, even if I am sure he knows what he is thinking and saying. Rafi's expression of desire and of faith often emerge in a way that is perplexing to us, in the form of deep, inarticulate sounds. They are mystifying words that are understood by God as he who hears even the unspoken. This is "the media of the Holy Spirit's intercession and they ascend to the throne of grace in the form of groanings."[2] Like Luke's multisensory approach to knowing, Paul presents us with a plurality of ways of communication.

For Paul, faith is hypocognitive. Faith lives under, beneath, or below the cognitive realm. Rafi's faith is a clear demonstration of this ideal. Unable to access words for certain concepts, he cannot communicate cognitive and linguistic representations. But despite his communication lacks, I have every confidence that the Holy Spirit has a full understanding of what is going on inside. God does not need us to have the "right" words and concepts.

Weakness and Flesh

It is in his letter to the church at Philippi that Paul sets out the fundamental dynamic that allows us to uncover the disability theology that runs through his thinking. Jesus voluntarily put himself at the bottom of the hierarchy, taking on the disability of servitude and crucifixion. In this Jesus makes common cause with the marginalized and the weak, in opposition to the glorification of power and authority that characterized the Roman Empire.

> Who, being in very nature God, did not consider equality with
> God something to be used to his own advantage; rather, he made

1. Murray, *Romans*, 312.
2. Murray, *Romans*, 312.

himself nothing by taking the very nature of a servant, being made in human likeness. And being found in appearance as a man, he humbled himself by becoming obedient to death—even death on a cross! Therefore, God exalted him to the highest place and gave him the name that is above every name, that at the name of Jesus every knee should bow, in heaven and on earth and under the earth, and every tongue acknowledge that Jesus Christ is Lord, to the glory of God the Father. (Phil 2:6–11)

For Paul, Christ is both disabled and glorified, weak and powerful, crucified and raised from the dead. Neither negates the other. One is not absorbed into the other, and the presence of one does not mean the absence of the other. "He was crucified because of weakness; He lives because of the power of God" (2 Cor 13:4). Christ is broken but lives again beyond disability and limitation, even the limitation of death. This paradox serves as the center of Paul's message, it is a dynamic that we are all invited into.

In Colossae, for example, Paul was almost certainly living in a filthy, hot, underground prison. He was chained together with others in crowded unsanitary rooms. The Roman strategy was to psychologically and physically torture, to strip prisoners of their dignity. He was probably anemic, malnourished, and utterly vulnerable. Paul had become a social non-entity.

I am now rejoicing in my suffering for your sake, and in my flesh, I am completing what is lacking in Christ's afflictions for the sake of his body, that is, the church. I became its servant according to God's commission that was given to me for you, to make the word of God fully known. (Col 1:24–25)

The word "suffering" can be understood as disability. I rejoice in my disability for your sake. Perhaps the "lack" here means to suggest that those to whom Paul proclaims the gospel are lacking in understanding of Christ's disability and death. Thus, when Paul suffers in this way, his listeners can see a model, albeit imperfect, of Christ's suffering and disability. Paul's own disability offers potential converts a persuasive portrayal of disability, in the pattern of the one who died to atone for them.

In Galatia, Paul was clearly in poor health. He needed care, housing, food. He might have needed help with hygiene and with dressing. His sickness was a responsibility to others.

As you know, it was because of an illness that I first preached the gospel to you, and even though my illness was a trial to you, you did not treat me with contempt or scorn. Instead, you welcomed

me as if I were an angel of God, as if I were Christ Jesus himself.
(Gal 4:13–14)

Some speculate that Paul might have in fact suffered from epilepsy, since he says in verse 14 that the Galatians did not treat him with contempt, a phrase that in could have connotations about demon possession from the physical manifestations of seizures. Some theorized that maybe he had contracted malaria. Whatever the cause of his illness, Paul would have needed support, and that required resources. But the community did not judge him for it, and he thanked them for accepting him and welcoming him despite his needs and the inconvenience associated with his incapacity.

The term "was a trial to you" is terse, indicating a negative—to spit out. To spit out was to avert evil influences or bad luck. Despite the possible social stigma or repulsion associated with sickness, or a cultural association between disability and sin, Paul commends them for not accepting this prevailing attitude. In accepting Paul's gospel, they accepted his weakness and saw the unity between the disabled Paul and the crucified, disabled Christ.

Paul encourages his readers to understand that God's purposes are fulfilled through our disabilities. God chooses to reveal disability so it might be abundantly clear that true ability is from God, "so that your faith might not rest on human wisdom, but on God's power" (1 Cor 2:5). In this way we might fully learn that all glory belongs exclusively to God, as Paul wrote: "But this happened that we might not rely on ourselves but on God, who raises the dead" (2 Cor 1:9).

The paradox is that Jesus' disability and weakness give us a life of ability and possibility. When we share in his disability, we share in his power. We overcome the disabilities that are revealed in our lives, our bodies, and our souls, by being in Christ:

- We always carry around in our body the death of Jesus, so that the life of Jesus may also be revealed in our body. (2 Cor 4:10)

- [W]e share in his sufferings in order that we may also share in his glory. (Rom 8:17)

- I want to know Christ—yes, to know the power of his resurrection and participation in his sufferings, becoming like him in his death. (Phil 3:10)

Paul regards himself as disabled, but this is the paradox of his ability, demonstrating God's power.

> I came to you in weakness with great fear and trembling. My message and my preaching were not with wise and persuasive words, but with a demonstration of the Spirit's power, so that your faith might not rest on human wisdom, but on God's power. (1 Cor 2:3–5)

For Paul, human disability reminds us of the power of God, the disability of Christ and a life that extends beyond disability and death. Paul describes Jesus (and us) as being at once disabled and powerful:

> For to be sure, he was crucified in weakness, yet he lives by God's power. Likewise, we are weak in him, yet by God's power we will live with him in our dealing with you. (2 Cor 13:4)

Jesus' humiliation in brokenness, disability, and weakness unlocks ability, power, and glory. "For if we have been united with him in a death like his, we will certainly also be united with him in a resurrection like his" (Rom 6:5).

Crucifixion was the ultimate stigma, a portrait of supreme weakness and suffering. As the antithesis of power, strength, and ability, Christ crucified is the definitive symbol of disability. It is on the cross that Christ shares and makes common cause with our disability and limitations, allowing his followers to participate in his suffering and receive atonement, thereby opening the way to a new life now and forever.

Paul's rich theological understanding also presents a challenge to the way that disability was commonly understood in the ancient Near East: it need not be related to stigma, sin, or demonic activity, but rather a genuine occasion to share in the power of the crucified and risen Christ.

Weakness is a reality that we all face. God disabuses us of the fact that we think we are strong. Eventually, one way or another, we will all be weak. There is no discrimination here. We are mortal and time grabs hold of us all. Sooner or later our capacities and health will decline, and we will need care.

But as followers in Christ, as for Paul, weakness can become more than just a reality that we reluctantly accept: it can become our vocation.

> For this light momentary affliction is preparing for us an eternal weight of glory beyond all comparison, as we look not to the things that are seen but to the things that are unseen. For the things that are seen are transient, but the things that are unseen are eternal. For we know that if the earthly tent we live in is destroyed, we have a building from God, an eternal house in heaven, not built by

human hands. Meanwhile we groan, longing to be clothed instead with our heavenly dwelling, because when we are clothed, we will not be found naked. For while we are in this tent, we groan and are burdened, because we do not wish to be unclothed but to be clothed instead with our heavenly dwelling, so that what is mortal may be swallowed up by life. Now the one who has fashioned us for this very purpose is God, who has given us the Spirit as a deposit, guaranteeing what is to come. (2 Cor 4:17–18; 5:1–5)

2 Corinthians: Paul's own Weakness as Vocation

Corinth was a challenging environment for Paul. It seems that competing philosophers came to the church displaying what some listeners felt to be a superior understanding. They were articulate and coherent, probably everything that Paul was not. Some believers challenged his authority as an apostle and criticized the way he spoke and presented himself: "His letters are weighty and forceful, but his bodily presence is weak, and his speech is contemptible" (2 Cor 10:10).

Paul's standing is impugned by pointing out his weaknesses. His body, his speech, and his whole person. The belief that character was evidenced by appearance was a prevalent one in the Greco-Roman world. Paul defends himself by radically reevaluating his disability. He begins by presenting standards he rejects:

> Whatever anyone else dares to boast about—I am speaking as a fool—I also dare to boast about. Are they Hebrews? So am I. Are they Israelites? So am I. Are they Abraham's descendants? So am I. (2 Cor 11:21–22)

Then Paul clearly lists his own experience of vulnerabilities and limitations, including hunger, imprisonment, beatings, and anxiety. But he is not ashamed of them: "If I must boast, I will boast of the things that show my weakness" (2 Cor 11:30).

> Therefore, in order to keep me from becoming conceited, I was given a thorn in my flesh, a messenger of Satan, to torment me. Three times I pleaded with the Lord to take it away from me. But he said to me, "My grace is sufficient for you, for my power is made perfect in weakness." Therefore, I will boast all the more gladly about my weaknesses, so that Christ's power may rest on me. (2 Cor 12:7–9)

Despite all this, Paul knows that his weakness makes him strong (2 Cor 12:10). We do not know for certain that this "thorn in his flesh" actually was, but we can imagine all sorts of unpleasantness or physical pain. Paul begs three times for this ailment to be removed from him, and while it remains, he comes to a sense of peace and wholeness together with that ailment.

Paul in fact defends his own limitations as something positive, as conduits for God's communication and evidence of God's power. This competitive world of gain and strength is now replaced by seeking to live in unity with Christ.

> We preach not ourselves, but Jesus Christ as Lord, and ourselves as your servants for Jesus' sake . . . we have this treasure in jars of clay to show that this all-surpassing power is from God and not from us. We always carry around in our body the death of Jesus, so that the life of Jesus may also be revealed in our body (2 Cor 4:5–6; 4:7–12)

Paul views his own disability as reflecting, in some sense, Jesus' death, and he sees in his own body evidence of Messiah's work. The conveyer of the message pictures the content of the message. As a result of this vivid portrayal, through Paul's experience of "death" by repeated disability, he delivers "the life of Jesus."

Second Corinthians 6:3–10 is foundational for understanding this dynamic.

> We put no stumbling block in anyone's path, so that our ministry will not be discredited. Rather, as servants of God we commend ourselves in every way: in great endurance; in troubles, hardships and distresses; in beatings, imprisonments and riots; in hard work, sleepless nights and hunger; in purity, understanding, patience and kindness; in the Holy Spirit and in sincere love; in truthful speech and in the power of God; with weapons of righteousness in the right hand and in the left; through glory and dishonor, bad report and good report; genuine, yet regarded as impostors; known, yet regarded as unknown; dying, and yet we live on; beaten, and yet not killed; sorrowful, yet always rejoicing; poor, yet making many rich; having nothing, and yet possessing everything.

The key concepts of weakness, suffering, and affliction reoccur in Paul's characterization of his ministry and himself. They seem to be set off by an additional set of key concepts, such as power, joy, and boasting. These two seemingly contradictory sets of concepts have a foundational bearing on how I see my own life, and Rafi's.

In verses 8–10 we have seven clauses introduced by the words "yet" or "as if." Paul is by no means suggesting that the challenges are not real. They are very real, and they are normal for any vocation to be carried out under these conditions. Being unknown, being weak and dying, in sorrow and in poverty: these are normal conditions. They serve to authenticate Paul's vocation as being Jesus-focused. We are not spiritual giants but broken men and women who lead others to the cross: the place of disability.

Paul is unique in the way he speaks about the brokenness of the human person and the fragility of our accomplishments. Nowhere has the disproportion between the task and the flimsiness of our equipment been more clearly presented. It seems that Paul's vocation is the weakest and least impressive human activity imaginable: the antithesis of a theology of power and glory.

In our day-to-day activities with Rafi, we wonder about the same sorts of things. Admittedly, we do not face the same life-threatening circumstances as did Paul. But I too wonder if I am known or an imposter. Does what we do make a difference? Is it phony? How do I posture myself? This profoundly affects my spirituality as caregiver. Rafi is utterly vulnerable as he receives care, but the more urgent question is my own vulnerability as an example and caregiver. Jesus became vulnerable and thus revealed sin. Had he been invulnerable, the true nature of sin would have stayed hidden. My own vulnerability needs to be transparent. Rafi needs to see me.

I have two choices when I ponder Rafi's weakness and mine. I can either use his condition as an excuse and not take responsibility for tending and helping and improving. Or I can confront his weakness and mine and plead for the strength and power to carry on.

I am forced every day to evaluate the values of the world that press in on me. "That is why, for Christ's sake, I delight in weaknesses, in insults, in hardships, in persecutions, in difficulties. For when I am weak, then I am strong" (2 Cor 12:10). Paul's words stand in stark contrast to the words in my face every day, of dividends, success, competition, achievement.

In Paul's view, God chooses to reveal himself through the weak and disabled of the world so that it might be clear that true power is from God alone. Yet human disabilities are not only a reminder that true power comes from God; they are also an occasion to participate in the disability and atoning death of Christ.

Concluding Thoughts on Paul and Difference

Paul's theory of disability disputes and corrects our world, which twists the truth about human power, ease, comfort, and ambition. There is a profound egocentricity in the desire for absolute sovereignty and mastery over ourselves, our bodies, and over the things of the world. The world is not perfectible, and some things cannot be fixed or mastered.

Paul presents us with a revolutionary way to think and to live. Rafi cannot be reconfigured. There is something divinely matchless about him, as there is about all of us. Rafi is, like many things, "unfixable, irresolvable, and definitive, just the way they are. God is the God of both sides of this conflict. Some honesty here would be in order."[3]

Ephraim Radner, who knows Rafi and has spent time with him, understands that we need to be honest about ability and disability and weakness. For Radner,

> resurrection is not the replacement of a life; it is a new life altogether, the divinely irreplaceable now made absolute for us. Thus, we always give thanks for what we have been given; and we pray for what is yet to be received in the fullness of glory. Holding both together, "His praise shall always be in my mouth" (Ps 34:1).[4]

The difference is to be found in the cross. How do we become disciples? Only through the cross, as Jesus says, "If any want to become my followers let them deny themselves and take up their cross and follow me" (Mark 8:34). The implication is that we all have a cross of our own to carry. We will all experience the disability, silence, aloneness, and abandonment of Jesus on the cross. How do we willingly accept this as part of our spirituality? How do we welcome this, not as failure but as a sign of true success?

In the world of our very real pain how could we worship a God who is immune to it? God suffered in Christ, but I think that God in Christ suffers with us, his people, still. God suffers with me, and I suffer as I care for Rafi. Jesus said that as we minister to the sick, the hungry, the naked, and the prisoner, we minister to him. He identifies with the needy and suffering today.

Christ suffered for us, and our sufferings are more manageable because of his. There remains a big question mark over suffering, but over it we can stamp another mark—the cross of Christ. This cross must be the

---

3. Radner, "Divine Irreplaceability."
4. Radner, "Divine Irreplaceability."

subject of our witness and the object of our boasting. We must come to terms with this vulnerability. Our functioning bodies and minds mask our inner world, and we fear this inadequacy. Is it possible to measure success in reflecting on and interpreting our own suffering and disability?

Rafi's day-to-day life is different than that of many, and he will always be a responsibility to others. He will always need care and help. His vocation is to be cared for in the body. But Rafi's vocation is not canceled out by his disability. It cannot be negated by bad health, pain, loss of memory, insults, or the cruelty of humanity or this world. For Paul, it is in brokenness that the glory of God is revealed, and to acknowledge one's imperfection does not encourage the romanticizing of flaws. The courage and willingness to face brokenness in the light of the power of the gospel became the main theme of his life.

Workbook Questions

1. Paul's theory of power is a radical one, for the ancient world and even today. Try to explain it in your own words. What is true power and where does it reside?

2. The author asserts that "weakness can become a vocation"—can you envision this? Write a paragraph outlining what this vocation might look like.

3. What are the implications of this vocation for thinking about limitations and disability?

10

Death and the Different

AN AVERAGE OF TEN people die by suicide each day in Canada. Ninety percent of these suicides are people living with a mental health problem or illness. As a result, in 2022 it was the thirteenth leading cause of death in Canada.[1]

Some 13,241 Canadians died via medically assisted death in 2022. From March 2027, mental illness alone, with no additional medical issue, will make a person eligible for assisted suicide in Canada. We do know that in 2022, 77.6 percent of MAID patients received palliative care. Some 63 percent had cancer and 17.1 percent of patients reported isolation or loneliness. Most requests for assisted death were due to pain and loss of autonomy.[2]

Euthanasia was legalized in Belgium in 2002, and in 2014 that law was expanded to include minors, regardless of their age. In Holland euthanasia is legal from the age of twelve and the law may be expanded to include younger children there as well.

Amniocentesis started being performed regularly in 1983. This test provides information about the fetus's genetic makeup. In the United States, there are reportedly 250,000 people with Down syndrome, and 45,000 in Canada. The termination rate for a fetus with Down syndrome is estimated at over 90 percent.[3]

1. See Canada Public Health Services, "Key Statistics" and "Suicide Prevention."
2. Health Canada, "Annual Report."
3. See Presson et al., "Current Estimate of Down Syndrome Population" for the

Iceland reports the disappearance of this condition in its country and Denmark is close behind.

A child born with Down syndrome in the USA needed a simple operation to repair an intestinal obstruction. The parents, a middle-income couple in their twenties, did not give permission. The infant died after fifteen days. A baby with Down syndrome was born with a malformed esophagus. The parents did not give permission to repair the defect and the hospital went to court. The Indiana Supreme Court voted to support the parents. The attorney for the parents called their decision "treatment to do nothing."[4]

A study was done of the withholding of care of handicapped infants in the Yale-New Haven Hospital. It was the breaking of a "public and professional silence on a major social taboo."[5]

Moral Reasoning and Human Action in Death

The moral issue of active death affects the disabled differently. I am especially mindful of the exceptional technological possibilities at our disposal today. Our ancestors coped without these choices, and we struggle under an illusion of control because of these many options. I want to reflect on the unimaginable new abilities we have—to manipulate, extend, and end life, and to relieve suffering and pain. This chapter is a meditation on suffering, mortality, technology, and disability.

After his bypass, my father was simply not motivated to get well. He deteriorated quickly and fought constantly with my exhausted mother. The hospice worker used words like "comfort" and "dignity" and "quality of life." It was euphemistic. My father died a few hours after being admitted to hospice care. I often wonder if a caring nurse checked him in and after looking at the chart gave him just enough morphine. It would have been a mercy and his passing probably saved my mother's life. Did the nurse need to use moral reasoning? Was my father's death active? He was eighty-six and overweight and had utterly given up.

United States, and Canadian Down Syndrome Society for Canada. See also Mansfield et al., "Termination."

4. Davis, *Evangelical Ethics*, 158.

5. Davis, *Evangelical Ethics*, 159.

My father never wanted the operation that he never recovered from. It involved six months of indignity and a major economic investment with no obvious benefit to my family.

The awesome power of medicine, in this situation, did more harm, and was deployed to extend a life that was ready to be over. In the same breath I marvel at the way medicine can diagnose and fix a fetus, the way that it can relieve tremendous human suffering. Medicine has this immense chance to offer consolation to the sick and suffering, but its mobilization demands rational limits. Its use for the disabled is even more complicated.

How do you bracket your own biases when making ethical decisions about active death when it comes to the different and disabled? I assert that you must examine all points of view and intentionally subject yourself to intensive proximity. We live in the real world, and the real world is full of particularity and specificity. I do not believe we can assert the same principle in all situations. And we can only know situations in any deep and true way through proximity.

Setting our preconceived notions aside and entering deeply and closely into a situation takes more time than most of us are willing to invest. We prefer simple absolutes and sound bites. But these are thin solutions to profound problems. We must think critically about how the relief of suffering is part of moral reasoning. How do we work out the commands of God in everyday life so that we form judgments that follow the way of Jesus? We must reflect on the extraordinary new abilities we have to manipulate, extend, and end life, and to relieve suffering and pain. How do we apply this to the disabled?

I grapple with the moral reasoning required around human suffering because of my experience with difference and disability. Our first obligation, in my view, is to seek out that proximity. This close immediacy will help us to enter deeply into the particulars of each person's story. It is only by exploring a person's life and honoring their humanity that we can begin to answer questions about morality and suffering. Each case is different, and each has a unique set of issues. We must become able to listen deeply and embrace ambiguity.

Because we are a culture of strangers, we are often forced to call unfamiliar, anonymous persons to this task. Medical professionals are strangers to us. They are too often not in close proximity. Do we really want them to read a chart and guide our decisions? It may be the worst day of our life, but for them it is another day at the office. Family and friends may be at a distance, too busy and distracted. How can we make these decisions when we are not in proximity and do not know deeply the particularity of one another's situation? I am reluctant to embrace an abstract principle and apply it to all cases in the same way. We have novel ethical problems, requiring us to consider courageously bracketing our principles for a time in certain instances. How should we think about the active hastening the end of a person's life? Some would assert that certain cases are morally ambiguous and that there is a positive moral duty to be humane.[6]

As an infant, Rafi suffered a collapsed lung. He was seen by a pulmonologist, several other doctors, therapists, and pediatricians, hooked up to machines that monitored him and delivered medicines. This treatment and therapy did the trick. We were sent home from the hospital within a few days with a supply of pills and puffers. What if Rafi had been born a hundred years ago to poor parents living in a poor country with no substantial resources? I remember reflecting on the utter weight of human suffering and the human dedication and ingenuity that we were able to benefit from.

I've written before that when I heard that Rafi had Down syndrome, I remember very clearly thinking that if I cannot handle this, my whole life, everything I stand for, is a lie. The thought still haunts me. What am I in all this—what kind of person do I want to be?

Proximity frees us from being attached to fears that can underlie our desire for clear absolutes. Being close to people and their specific situations engages all our reasoning and demands the courage to listen to people in their unique physical, social, emotional, and economic sufferings. It is about people, not about principles. Our presuppositions and abstract morality is like a finger resting on the balance scales, giving us biased and inaccurate results.

Technology gives the illusion of control, both giving and taking away in ways that previous generations could never have imagined. Medicine can end life quickly and it can prolong life. Visiting my father in the cardiac ward was hellish: a few rooms with near-dead people and an enormous number of medical professionals and machines working to keep those people alive. After a few days of chatting, I asked the doctor how he comes to work every day. He just smiled. I wonder what kind of defense mechanisms he has in place.

I imagine that our ancestors encountered death quite regularly from close-up. Today we see it hardly at all. Until recently, people only rarely

6. Kohl, "Beneficent Euthanasia."

lived beyond their forties. Many mothers and children died in childbirth. People often died at home, known to family and friends. Today our life expectancy has doubled, and we live in neighborhoods of strangers. We do not live with our (grown) children or parents and so there is no sense of generational continuity, care, or death. Increasingly we depend on an impersonal government to decide and deploy its resources to help and bring care. The care comes in shifts and is delivered by strangers. Ambulances take the sick and dying away to some other place.

Moral Reasoning

A devout Catholic, Dr. John Rock graduated from Harvard Medical School in 1918. Over his many years practicing obstetrics in Boston, he witnessed firsthand the suffering endured by women from multiple pregnancies: collapsed wombs, premature aging, and financial despair.

His patients' experiences weighed heavily on him. Rock was not interested in dogmatic reform at all, but rather he came to see the use of artificial birth control within marriage as a means of alleviating human suffering. He believed in the power of birth control to reduce poverty and prevent illness. Alleviation of unnecessary human suffering was the principle that guided him to help invent oral contraception. He asserted that oral contraception was a natural extension of the rhythm method. He argued it was the way of Jesus. His beliefs arose out of the proximity to human suffering, an experience that changed his approach to moral reasoning.

Rock wanted to honor the sanctity of life and the moral position of the church, but at the same time he felt that one could not begin with abstract principles. Rock's moral reasoning began with the particularities of the situation and derived from a deep understanding of the problem. His abstract principles were grounded in the specifics. Rock found himself unable to offer platitudes in the face of human suffering, and he believed his was the way of the gospel.[7]

Questions about human suffering and the cost of care are worthy ones. Jewish and Christian witness is to be realistic in our acknowledgment of the suffering that comes with disability. There is a concrete reality to the permanent financial and emotional burdens that disability inflicts upon those who care. There are also tangible costs to the communities we live in. Local hospitals do not have infinite resources. There is also very real

7. Gladwell, "John Rock's Error."

physical and emotional suffering among the disabled. How do we alleviate suffering and provide care? Where do the resources come from? The burdens that disability leaves in its wake must include the vulnerability and limitations of both those who care and of those who are cared for.

In a 2014 response to a woman who tweeted about the predicament of knowing her baby would be born with Down syndrome, ethicist Richard Dawkins replied, "Abort it and try again. It would be immoral to bring it into the world."[8] When his statement was met with public outrage, Dawkins tried to modify things: "To conclude, what I was saying simply follows logically from the ordinary pro-choice stance that most of us, I presume, espouse. My phraseology may have been tactlessly vulnerable to misunderstanding, but I can't help feeling that at least half the problem lies in a wanton eagerness to misunderstand."[9]

"Speciesism" is a term popularized by moral philosopher Peter Singer to describe the way that humans give less weight to the interests of nonhuman animals than they give to human beings. Singer does not think it is "specieist" to believe that humans are more important than animals in certain circumstances. He maintains however that it is speciesism to say human life is always more important, a belief that allows him to also assert that some infants with severe disabilities should be killed:

> When the death of a disabled infant will lead to the birth of another infant with better prospects of a happy life, the total amount of happiness will be greater if the disabled infant is killed. The loss of a happy life for the first infant is outweighed by the gain of a happier life for the second. Therefore, if killing the hemophiliac infant has no adverse effect on others, it would, according to the total view, be right to kill him.[10]

Moral Reasoning and Suicide

Suicide has always alarmed me. When I have heard of friends or acquaintances who have actively killed themselves, it takes my breath away. Artists and entertainers who have touched me over the years in one way or another and who have committed suicide cause me to pause. Ernest Hemingway

8. Press Association, "Richard Dawkins."
9. Press Association, "Richard Dawkins."
10. Singer, *Practical Ethics*, 186.

judged his father for his own suicide, but eventually the clouds of agonizing depression descended on him as well. He was ill and sought and received care at one of the best hospitals in the world. But the pain was too great, and he needed the relief that alcohol and medical therapies could not provide. That relief could only come at his own hand.

Antiquity saw extensive philosophical debates about suicide. Both suicide and euthanasia were often seen as a good way to die, a means of deliverance from affliction and oppression. In general, ancient society did not attach any disgrace to the practice, provided there was sufficient justification.

Traditionally the faithful see voluntary death as a case of usurping God's powers. Some say the act is cowardly and selfish. God has given life to humans and God alone has the right to take it away. He asks us to be ready for death at every moment. Who has the right to determine when or how we leave?

Suicide can be a failure of medicine. Suicide can be a sign of failure of community. This is especially cogent in our society where the pursuit of life, liberty, and happiness is often confused with autonomy and hallowed by the ethics of individualism. Perhaps within this kind of ethic we do have the right to commit suicide.

When I saw the news of Robin Williams's suicide, I was gut-punched. He gave me hours of entertainment and the simple pleasure of silliness and laughter. I had been to his concerts and seen his movies and read that he was kind and generous and charitable. He expressed love and affection for his family and friends and at the same time he was a drug and alcohol addict wrestling with depression. He seemed open about this struggle, and I am sure fans who were similarly afflicted drew comfort from the support.

I wondered what depression felt like. Does it have texture and composition? How does it hurt? The relationship between the suicidal act and its context seems to be central to our problem. Some place the act itself in principal position. Others will give context the primary position. Williams was gifted and tormented. The torment fed his gift, and his gift could not release his torment. He was obviously sick, in pain and afraid. Did his community fail him? Did he lack the courage to be a witness to his community? Was he afraid of being cared for?

I wonder about people who lived under regular conditions of deprivation: prisoners of war, slaves, the poor and the homeless. Eugene Genovese, an American historian of slavery and the American South, showed in this research that:

> Even though we often think of suicide occurring under conditions of extreme stress or constant threat of life; slaves never committed suicide in large numbers; though abandoned by the white society, they found a sustaining faithfulness in their own community. The assertion that slaves frequently committed suicide, quaintly put forward by some historians as a form of "day-to-day resistance to slavery," rests on no discernible evidence. The strong sense of stewardship in the quarters—of collective responsibility for each other—probably accounts for the low suicide rate more than does any other factor.[11]

There is something about proximity to different generations that provides some of the hope and sustenance that motivates us to endure. The sense of memory provided by story offers strength and consolation. Living together generationally provides structure of this memory. Even in times of deprivation, some of the bewilderment of pain will be blunted by the harmony, consistency, and power of the story of which you are a part.

King Saul, after being defeated by the Philistines, realized what would happen to him if he were captured alive. To prevent this, Saul impaled himself on his own sword (1 Sam 31:4). According to Jewish law, there is a differentiation that must be made between people who are in full possession of their physical and mental facilities and those people who act on impulse or who are under severe mental or physical duress.

Jewish law speaks of an individual in this second category of being a "person under compulsion," and not responsible for his actions. Many authorities of subsequent generations have ruled that most suicides are to be considered as having acted under compulsion when taking their own lives. As such, they are not responsible for their actions and are to be accorded the same courtesies and privileges granted a Jew who has met a natural death.

Euthanasia and Moral Reasoning

At the beginning of the twentieth century, the sterilization of people carrying what were felt to be hereditary defects and "antisocial" behavior was a respectable medical practice. The West passed laws enabling coerced sterilization. In 1927 the United States Supreme Court upheld the

---

11. Genovese, *Roll, Jordan, Roll*, 639–40.

constitutionality of involuntary sterilization of individuals with mental retardation. In the decision, Judge Oliver Wendall Holmes stated that

> it is better for all the world if instead of waiting to execute degenerate offspring for crime or to let them starve for their imbecility, society can prevent those who are manifestly unfit from continuing their kind . . . Three generations of imbeciles are enough.[12]

Studies conducted in the 1920s showed Germany as a country that was unusually reluctant to introduce sterilization legislation. But in *Mein Kampf* (1924), Adolf Hitler wrote that one day racial hygiene "will appear as a deed greater than the most victorious wars of our present [. . .] era." Propaganda posters began appearing showing the disabled as multiplying out of control and threatening to overwhelm German society.

Hitler wrote this directive on September 1, 1939:

> Reich Leader Bouhler and Dr. Brandt are entrusted with the responsibility of extending the authority of physicians, to be designated by name, so that patients who, after a most critical diagnosis, on the basis of human judgment are considered incurable, can be granted mercy death.[13]

This euphemistically designed memo seems to have been the beginning of the end for the disabled in Germany. Action T4 was the postwar name given for mass murder by involuntary euthanasia in Nazi Germany. Estimates are that some 275,000 to 300,000 disabled victims were euthanized during the war. Economic rationalities and racial purity were the central factors in the devaluing of people with disabilities.

Stanley Hauerwas's insights are most trenchant here:

> Euthanasia is often supported by the most humane arguments [and] cannot not become a way of doing away with those who bother us rather than giving them care. It may be that the demand for euthanasia comes because we lack the skills humanly to know how to be with and care for the dying, especially when we are the one doing the dying. Humans never kill more readily than when we kill in the name of mercy. We must be careful that the mercy we dispense, especially when it takes the form of ending life, is

---

12. *Buck v Bell*, 274 U.S. 2000, 1927.

13. The signed memo authorizing Aktion T4 can be found at https://ghdi.ghi-dc.org/sub_document.cfm?document_id=1528. It is widely understood to have been written in October of 1939 and backdated to September 1, 1939.

not necessary because of our original uncare. . . . The pathogenic abandonment of the individual by his or her community is the final affirmation and sealing of a long process of abandonment by the community, the dramatic expression of an abandonment experienced across a person's lifetime.[14]

Mortality

From our conception we are subject to death. To number our days is to take seriously our mortality: this must be our point of entry to moral reasoning about active death and will help us to figure out our lives and how we engage with others and with God. It is foundational in discussing death and the disabled.

We all have bodies that will succumb. We are not permanent, and we cannot look to the world for permanence. I don't think that people in the modern West think about this reality too often, but we really ought to. We assume that the power of medicine will keep this fact at bay. We do not want proximity to death, but that proximity will change how we reason morally about the grave questions we face.[15]

The increase in life expectancy and the reduction in infant mortality in the last century have changed how we think about living and dying. It has changed how we think about our bodies and what we do with them, irrespective of our status as normally developing or disabled or different. Our ancestors saw death as something of a gift that was inevitable and expected. They knew that we are fragile, mortal, yet somehow glorious. We see death as something else—what Radner calls "a wrecking ball."[16]

We avoid death by living disconnected from our older generations. I grew up in a multigenerational home with another generation just a short drive away. My grandmother's decline into dementia was a turning point in my adolescence. She lived with us and then with my aunt's family. It was heartbreaking to watch things be taken from her. This was a woman who sailed to America from Poland in 1904 at the age of fourteen, without a word of English. This person was reduced to wearing diapers and staring out a window all day. My proximity to her decline and death continues

14. Hauerwas, *Hauerwas Reader*, 591.

15. Radner, *Time to Keep*. My discussions with Dr. Radner, and this book, have been very helpful in guiding me through these issues.

16. Radner, "Psychedelic Body."

to affect the way I think about my own humanity and my limitations. I should have helped bathe her and clean her and toilet her and feed her. I was ashamed to volunteer, and I was never asked. The care almost broke our family, but it should not have.

I was a teenager during her decline, having just completed a rigorous time of religious education culminating in my Bar Mitzvah. I was busy thinking more about girls than about my grandmother or God. But then I saw her, and I thought for the first time about her as a human being. To whom did her body belong? It did not seem to belong to her anymore. I realized that we persist as profoundly limited beings.

I remember my parents fighting with other family members about my grandmother's care and about money. It was fracturing our family. This went on for two years. Her death was a tragedy and a mercy. As I think about it from this safe point of view, it should have been a time when we all cared together. When I take care of Rafi in that kind of way, I often think of her. How do we prepare on the safe side of all this before urgent care is needed? I think it has something to do with living generationally in proximity to difference.

Mortality cannot not be circumvented. If we are God's and life is wholly a gift from him, then mortality if a gift from him as well. The constraints that mortality imposes should be honored. My faithfulness to my own mortality and to Rafi's mortality is to take care of myself and him. This seems the proper response to the gift of my temporal limitation and Rafi's. As I do this I recognize and then accept life's limitations and I try to be faithful without resentment. I am not escaping or denying. This is my body, and this is Rafi's body. It is what we have and there is nothing else.

Different people will have different stories, but no one exists cut off from the reality of mortality. If we have no convictions about mortality, our culture will provide them for us. If our convictions are poorly understood or weakly held, prevailing cultural patterns will take precedence. If you are never in proximity to death, difference, or disability, how will your story have convictions? You can speak articulately and intelligently and argue forcefully, but will your story resonate with the different and the disabled? When those convictions are based on proximity, you can return to and find continual recourse in the sources of the strength of convictions.

For Christians, the reasons for living begin with the understanding that life is a gift, we are mortal, and we have a vocation. We are not our own creators. Our desire to live should be shaped in the affirmation that we are not the determiners of our life, but God is. We are part of a bigger story and there is nothing wrong with being a burden. It is the vocation of being cared for by those who provide care. The care of the dying and the disabled is an essential act for witnessing our celebration of their lives and ours. This story is our testimony to the world.

When J. R. R. Tolkien asserts that divine punishments and pain are also divine gifts, I think he was reflecting on what we cannot get around: it is a gift to exist, and with that comes suffering, and the disabled are part of that gifting to the world.

> What is given is not ours to dispose of as if we created it, nor ours to use to serve only our own interests, to mutilate, wantonly destroy, and to deprive others of. Rather, if life is given in grace and freedom and love, we are to care for it and share it graciously, freely and in gratitude to him we have reason enough to seek the good of others and are moved to do so.[17]

There are different ways of dying. When the time comes for us to be cared for, we have at our disposal ways that our ancestors never knew. How do we deploy that care? Our ancestors' lives were short and often painful. Today we are involved in discussions that suggest we should be able to determine when our own life will end and what we shall do with it.

My own position is that our lives are formed in terms not of what we will do with them, but of what God will do with our lives, both in our living and our dying. It is our duty to care and to be cared for. At the same time, while life is sacred, I wonder if we must in fact hold on to it to the last minute. Life is not an absolute and I do not think that God wants us to place unwarranted value on it.

The apostle Paul accepted the fate of his ending as a way of affirming the trustworthiness of God's care for him. He would not fight death when it could not be avoided. "For I am already being poured out like a drink offering, and the time for my departure is near. I have fought the good fight, I have finished the race, I have kept the faith" (2 Tim 4:6–7).

We need a language of finitude and mortality. We need a way of speaking decently about the limits of human life. We need a way of saying why and under what circumstances death is natural. This language would not deny that early death or painful death are matters we wish to avoid. We need to know that our purpose is not unconditional existence.

The Hebrew Bible consoles us here:

17. Gustafson, *Theology and Christian Ethics*, 170.

From everlasting to everlasting, you are God. A thousand years in your sight are like a day that has just gone by. Yet you sweep people away in the sleep of death—Our days may come to seventy years, or eighty, if our strength endures; for they quickly pass, and we fly away. Teach us to number our days, that we may gain a heart of wisdom. Relent, Lord! How long will it be? Satisfy us in the morning with your unfailing love, that we may sing for joy and be glad all our days. Make us glad for as many days as you have afflicted us, for as many years as we have seen trouble. May your deeds be shown to your servants, your splendor to their children. (Ps 90:2; 4–5; 10; 12–16)

How does this help? It reminds us that God is God and we are not. Life is temporary, but he is not. Satisfaction will not take place in this world. Each day and all that it brings is a gift. Those who come after will remember us and our stories. This helps to answer questions about story and memory and death. "Presence" is the fundamental meaning of memory.

Taking the life of the disabled eradicates the presence of these people and results in their loss in our memory. Their existence—their presence in our lives—has moral importance that we must notice. In the same manner, we know we must be here and be willing to die in a way that makes it possible for us to be present in the memory of others. Any death provides an opportunity to speak to the world. The world celebrates choice, but this is one thing we cannot choose. The problem of death persists and cries out for an answer. If death exists, people will ask about the meaning of life. As death approaches, the noise of the world subsides. People become more willing to listen and think at this time.

Life is fragile, and death is devastating. These are two biblical truths that we need to place at the heart of the conversation of active death of the different and disabled. Why does death hurt? Why does it provoke lament? Why is the passing of a loved one different from the falling of an autumn leaf? Because it is a deprivation of the present, and that which has existed has been torn away. The death of a person with a history, and the more that history has shaped who we are in the present, the more the death deprives us of our future. A little piece of us has died with the death of another, whether a child who emerges stillborn, the disabled, or a grandparent. We are diminished and this is a deprivation of our being, painful and permanent. I hope that Rafi's death will bring all that because his life was filled with history.

My revulsion toward suicide, euthanasia, and abortion is a way of affirming how we should die in our communities in a nondestructive way for those that continue after us. It is a symbolic claim that insists that we remember our primary business is about living, not dying. A moral prohibition is not meant to point a judgmental finger. It is meant to awaken us to the convictions needed to shape the character of our communities. Can we honor life and alleviate suffering?

Concluding Thoughts on Death and the Different

In Clint Eastwood's popular movie *Million Dollar Baby*, the hero is a young boxing champion. After enduring a terrible accident she is left a quadriplegic and later undergoes the amputation of one leg. When she asks her friend and mentor to end her life, her argument is simple: "I met my goals, I am satisfied, this is a waste, I am at peace, and my life is a celebration." He eventually euthanizes her.

The film received a great deal of criticism from the disability community for its thin portrayal of disability. The complaint against the film's portrayal of euthanasia grew out of this absence of proximity even though the person who took her life in the movie was deeply proximate. This was the complaint:

> They are dealing in the grand myths and legends that surround the idea of disability rather than the reality of living with a disability . . . Few people have personal experience with severe disabilities, and few will take the time to find out about what life is like living with deafness, blindness or disability.[18]

A request to end the life of a suffering or disabled person invites us to be part of a story that we might not want to be in, to be a part of another person's determination whether they should live or die. In *Million Dollar Baby*, the man finds himself in proximity to real pain and suffering and hopelessness. What seemed like a reasonable request moved him to act. He saw it as a terrible mercy and the filmmakers encourage us to think that way as well. The film is asking us to join in his proximity and think about how that would change you.

If we are to learn to look on life as a gift, then any care is a symbolic act of the trustworthiness of our existence. When we allow others to care

18. *Chicago Tribune*, "Why 'Million Dollar Baby' infuriates."

we are saying something about trust. Where does our authority lie in such matters? If our vocation is to care, then is the alleviation of suffering part of that care? Living often requires courage to endure. This position involves assumptions about the moral role of suffering.

Suffering is not an evil to overcome but a part of life we must learn to live with. This suffering is relative and temporary, we should be willing to bear it for the good and with the aid of the community. This is for us and others so we will not put ourselves, our friends and family in the position of wanting to die. Some might fear boredom and uselessness even more than suffering. Is it our right to end life prematurely because we fear boredom?

The distinction between "putting to death" and "letting die" makes sense to me. The moral reasoning not to actively intervene, but rather to refrain from acting, is to show the one who suffers the continuing credibility of his or her existence in a body.

Autonomy in dying, as in living, is often considered the mark of being free, unhindered, and self-supporting. Rafi lives in dependence but not without dignity. He has meaningful involvement in the lives of others and enjoys a robust range of encounters. Rafi has a zeal for life. Even his sadness and anxieties and limitations help me to discover the unique significance of those who are most vulnerable in our world.

Workbook Questions

1. The author embraces the value of proximity as an essential piece of moral reasoning. Think about a time when you been truly proximate to another person's suffering.

2. What might make us hesitate to embrace this kind of proximity?

3. Consider your own experiences of death. Has it been avoided or accepted? Scrubbed clean or engaged closely?

11

Difference in Sexuality

A FAMILY SHOWED UP to a local church. They were a spiritually hungry lesbian couple and two children. They came faithfully to worship and eventually told the elders that they wanted to put their faith and hope in Jesus and live in Christ. They came forward for baptism. Interviewing showed that this was a stable family living in the community, sincere in their commitment and holding no agenda. After much hand-wringing the elders wanted to request that the couple divorce as a condition of baptism. About to call the family with this news, the pastor realized the absurdity of this position. He baptized them all and welcomed them into the church just like any other persons of faith.

Rafi is a twenty-six-year-old man. He will not have a sexual life of any kind. I would guess that he might have sexual thoughts, but I am not sure how he reflects on and processes them. I can tell that he likes girls. He sometimes gets physically aroused but I do not think he has an awareness of what we could call his "sexuality." Nudity is completely neutral to Rafi.

I wonder if he is frustrated because he cannot express himself sexually. I know that some people with Down syndrome do marry and some are sexually active, but Rafi does not seem to have the facility for that kind of intimacy. He enjoys both men and women as friends and companions. If Rafi did turn out to have the capacity for marriage, I think I would be delighted. The immediacy of his difference has provoked in me a new way of thinking about human difference in sexuality.

When I think about human difference and sexuality, I think about my own heterosexuality. I also think of all the people I know who are different than me in their sexuality. I think about limits, margins, and boundaries. I often wonder if there is any moral difference for those who are sexually active and covenanted with a consenting adult. I believe that God is the just judge of all the earth, and I assert that certain behavior falls outside the limits of moral behavior. But I am also deeply concerned with the matter of the vows and commitments we make to one another, the ones we make to God, and those he makes to us.

Obviously the sexually different are not disabled, but my convictions about proximity are the same. We are impoverished if we are not in proximity to those who are different, and that includes proximity to those with a different form of sexuality.

Proximity and Moral Reasoning

I'd like this chapter to be engaging and challenging to readers who are willing to think further with me. I don't want to get into a hermeneutical brawl. I don't want the conversation to devolve into a slippery slope of deviant and illegal behaviors that are beyond my understanding of the different. I don't claim to have a perfect understanding of the truth. Most LGBT people who are outside the church, it seems to me, just want to get on with their lives as well. My focus here is on covenanted people. My personal convictions are these: certainly the scriptural proscriptions are severe. Yet I do not believe that covenanted and/or monogamous people who are sexually different should be bound by this prohibition if they are in a covenanted relationship. I have gay friends and family who are serious about God, and the cliché of accepting but not affirming is really neither. There needs to be a wiser way of dealing with this. I think that the difference in male and female bodies is important, foundational even, but I do not see an appeal to creation as proscriptive. Rather, I see the creation story as descriptive of difference. I want to be a generous man of faith. I believe that God is the true judge, not me. Labels encourage us to give up thinking for ourselves. I want gay people to be accepted and included and most importantly to belong to God and his people. Sexually different people must belong in the work of God and be made to know this through welcome and inclusion, in the same way that Rafi should belong. I don't want to imply that people who are sexually different are in any way disabled, but the principles of respect, dignity, and belonging are the same for me. My convictions about sexual difference flow out of my proximity to Rafi.

When I use the word "covenant," it might be religious or nonreligious. But it I mean "committed" to a person, as one might be committed to God. The bottom line for me is that I want people to deal with issues of purity like I do—before God. I want them to know Jesus the King of Israel and I want them to put their hope and trust in him. I have written of my cousin and others that I know who are sexually different and how I want them to be covenanted. When people are covenanted in communities to God and one another, then God works.

These convictions might strike some as tangential to the rest of the book. They are not. They are an integral part of entire theology of difference. This chapter is not peripheral.

Theological Reflection

Are the proscriptions against homosexual behavior that we see in the biblical text transcultural, and do they apply for covenanted people? This is the problem I need to grapple with. I would agree that Scripture is interested in purity but the text strikes me as rather more focused on sins of covetousness, lust, gluttony, envy, anger, sloth, greed, and presumption, while sexual proscriptions are often contexted in the idolatrous behavior of the nations. Did the ancient writers even imagine that an orientation towards homosexuality was an option that could be considered within the covenant? It seems like an argument from silence. The ancients did not do particularly well with difference.

Once in Eastern Europe I was training a large group of church leaders on ways to address particular difficult, taboo subjects. When I asked them if they had ministry among people who were gay, one pastor stood up and asserted "we don't have that problem here." I asked how many in the group had been in the church where I spoke the previous day, and many raised their hands. I told them that there must have been ten to fifty people in that church of a thousand whose sexual orientation was different.

In this country where I found myself, I knew that local laws that criminalize homosexuality create a self-fulfilling prophecy. Just because you cannot see it does not mean it is not there. In that country, people who are sexually different risk their freedom, their lives, and their vocations. I told them that these people are in your families and communities, and they need and deserve compassion and inclusion. I told them that you cannot argue with human difference. It is part of being normal.

Many of the listeners were upset. But some came up to me afterwards and admitted that they knew people who were gay. As the days moved on, I think the group grew to respect my desire to open the conversation even in disagreement. That was my hope. Time and proximity have a way of working things out.

I want to try to think reasonably and morally situate myself with particular LGBTQ people and temporarily bracket out abstract principles and presuppositions. I think that concepts like "disordered attachments" are like a finger on the scale, and that proximity to real and particular difference can free you from being attached to fear. I want to get out of the way of my own biases and be open and free to listen to the lives, feelings, challenges, and hopes of those who live with difference. When I make a moral reasoning on this issue, I do not want to do so as a stranger. We must situate ourselves closely, listen deeply. We have an obligation to offer consolation to the suffering: this is what people of faith do.

I want to approach this problem on its own and to begin with an effort to understand the specifics and nature of the problem. If we advance from the particulars, then we can consider new kinds of problems on their own merits so that clear moral direction can be taken and consolation offered without in any way contradicting a principled position.

I want to honor the sanctity of the human body as belonging to God and respect the moral position of the church on the sacredness of sexual relationships. But we must have more to offer than just platitudes. I believe this was the way of the gospel. I want to think well about mortality, humanity, and our own limitations, about hope for the future, and caring and being cared for in what can be a short and sometimes tragic life.[1] I want to think properly about what is means to be a human being.

When I meet monogamous and faithful LGBTQ Christians, I first see an overwhelming association of similarity and familiarity on all these important questions. I also see my own brokenness.

---

1. See Radner, *Time to Keep*. This book is invaluable. Radner argues that mortality should not be resisted but acknowledged as a gift to be received. The limitations that mortality imposes should be celebrated. Resignation, escape, and denial are not appropriate responses to the gift of life and mortality. Faithfulness is the proper response to the gift of humanity's temporal limitation. To live rightly is to recognize and then willingly accept life's limitations imposed by mortality.

Some years ago, I was in the Castro district in San Francisco, a neighborhood well known as a center of LGBTQ history and activism. When I saw a male couple walking down the street with a young man who had Down syndrome, I took my phone out and showed the couple a picture of Rafi. They were thrilled. I asked if they would mind a couple of questions. They were open and refreshingly immediate and friendly. They told me that since same-sex marriage had been legalized they wanted to adopt children together, but the only children that were available to adopt were older and had special needs. This young man was their first child, and they were planning a second adoption of a young girl with Down syndrome. We chatted for a few minutes, and they asked about Rafi and how he was doing, and they asked me some questions about public policy and disability benefits in Toronto. As I walked home, I was thinking about the neighborhood where these two young people with Down syndrome were going to grow up. I imagined what life would be like for Rafi in the Castro with its inner-city feel, apartments, and comfortable vibe. Later that week I took a short drive across the Golden Gate Bridge to Marin County, which has the sixth highest income per capita of all US counties. I thought about what Rafi's life would be like in Marin. I thought about which neighborhood Rafi would find the most acknowledgment, inclusion, and enablement. Both areas are demographically similar. Where would his difference be most welcome and accepted? I think of this Castro district family often.

Male and Female

The biblical pronouncement "He created them male and female" is descriptive: a statement of human difference. It is also a statement of human dignity. Genesis shook the ancient world with a bold claim that all people are made in the image of God. That was, and remains, revolutionary. This dignity means that each human person has intrinsic honor and worth. Nowhere is the image of God defined explicitly, but it is described in the accounts of Genesis 1 and 2. The true distinguishing characteristic of human beings, as distinct from other creatures, is the purpose for which God has created us. To be sexually different is not the loss or diminishment of personhood, vocation, or dignity. Genesis is descriptive of the supremacy of the heterosexual act, but not an absolute prescription. We see that all humanity that comes from male and female is made in the image of God.

I see those who are different as having an orientation that is funda-mental to who they are in the image of God, and thus to their dignity. Most people would agree that the presence of sexual desire is a natural one and that sexuality is first a predisposition and only then a choice. I myself can-not remember ever *not* being attracted to women: it is how I was created. This predisposition does not mean, however, that there are no limits. The way that difference behaves, must, just as all human behavior, be defined by coherent limits. I assert that it is proper that there should be inherent and sensible limits on sexual activity. At the same time, we live in the real world of difference. We need to create space for difference to exist with dignity and without fear. We see this in the laws protecting strangers. The Hebrew Bible speaks of this in a subversive way. God's power is made known in the stranger's lack of ability, his need and his vulnerability, not in his autonomy or power. When we come to own our limitations and vulnerabilities, we are not averse to human difference.

I ask myself: "How can I deny LGBTQ couples what I have—the bless-ings of covenanted marriage in the eyes of God—if that is what they seek?" I should want to include and approve and be part of unions like these, ones based in commitment, monogamy, companionship, and the quest for holi-ness. I should actively reach out and support such families, those who want to be or can be reached, so that they can be covenanted.

There is both the value of covenant and commitment and there is the gospel, which requires surrender and submission to the God of Israel and his Messiah Jesus. My desire is for all couples to experience both, but the minimum is the first. If that kind of covenanted relationship is possible in the context of a LGBTQ relationship (or any number of heterosexual rela-tionships that might be considered problematic) then that is the place to start. We must reach out to comfort and include all those who are margin-alized, who may think they are accidents, mistakes, or broken by virtue of their difference. This is true for both the disabled and the sexually differ-ent. For these people it must be terribly destructive to hear constantly that they must be healed in a way different from the healing that all humans need. Let us be in proximity to this essential desire that all people have, to be in relationship.

Homosexuality is simply another form of human difference, and proximity to difference transforms both parties. I absolutely assert that sex is sacred: I insist that our bodies belong to God, and we are accountable to God for how we use them. Foundational to our purpose as humanity is our ability to create new generations of males and females. This is sacred as well. I also think that covenanted, accountable, monogamous sexuality can exist for those who are gay. Just because they cannot create new biological generations does not make their relationships less than sacred. For me, it is the vow that changes everything. People can be different, but their vows can be the same. How to honor the dignity of the real people that we know, gay men and women who are living out the Christian life, who are committed to the work of God and who are in relationships that seek to honor the God of Israel and the Messiah Jesus.

Sexual ordering must be normatively heterosexual because it is essential for procreation and survival. Yet it is also the case that some are different, and some cannot and will not be able to fit inside a generational passage. People can agree that sexuality is important beyond immediate indulgence, but that it is also valuable beyond its procreative potential.

My responsibility is not to condemn or reject people who are sexually different, but to endeavor to draw them into fellowship with the God of Israel and Jesus Christ. This is consistent with my feelings about all human difference. To call homosexual orientation disordered is itself disordered, and as wrong as calling the disabled a mistake or an accident. What is Jesus calling us to do among the stranger, the disabled, and any despised people in the world? These are also the frightened and the bullied, the rejected and the suicidal. Like Rafi, they need to be protected, given space, encouraged, and heartened to experience the love of God in Messiah.

Thick or Thin: Disabled and Homosexual

Homosexuality is not a neutral term. It is deeply theological, social, and anthropological. We are talking about people with families and commitments, lives and hopes. A thin description will not do, just as I cannot accept thin descriptions of Rafi. Rafi is a twenty-six-year-old man who has a life, friends, family, work, and a future. Down syndrome is a feature of that, of course, but he must not be defined that way. Any term that sums up human difference without reference to the unique individual is troubling. What is life is like for the different and what does it mean to belong? We live in a thin world. Rafi is known and loved and appreciated, but nothing else. He is not included, and he does not fully belong. Do we do the same to our gay family and friends?

People who are different, sexually and otherwise, will increasingly be in proximity to us as family and co-workers, friends and congregants. The classical response, that you "accept but do not affirm" is received as neither. If people assert that they feel the liberty of the Holy Spirit to live in a covenanted gay relationship, who am I to say, as a fundamentally broken person, that this difference is disordered or not normal?

What is normal? The norm is to be different. Thick approaches demand drilling down to individual situations and choosing limits carefully. Can we celebrate human difference with limits? The Christian tradition usually sees many ways as normal. I have lived in many places and have met many kinds of people who worship and hear and understand Scripture and humanity very differently. The norm is difference and plurality.

The church should be the last place to be surprised by human difference. Difference cannot be washed away in a tide of normalcy. Normalcy cannot be ritualized in the body of Christ. We do not need a common norm but a community that enables sacred limits. I am not separate and superior, and I cannot divide people into opposite categories and ascribe value to them of good and bad or higher and lower. I can only encourage them to be in covenant and submit to the authority of God and his word as I would all people.

I see both sides. I see the ugliness in broken people and broken sexuality. I have no romantic illusions. God's grace comes into our brokenness, with a goodness that surprises and refreshes. He calls us to love the stranger and the marginal, and yet much of our tradition forbids homosexual relationships and condemns the institutionalization of such relationships as marriages. There is a good instinct at work when we appeal to nature and to creation in our traditions. It is rooted in the norm, and without norms we would dissolve. I aspire to a coherent view of difference, but difference is not a disorder—it is simply difference.

Concluding Thoughts on Difference in Sexuality

We can be orthodox and at the same time be generous and listen carefully to people who are sexually oriented in a different way. To stand on orthodoxy, without reference and regard to particular individuals and their specific lives, seems superficial and hollow. This is about the gospel and following the way of Jesus. It is about living out our faith in the real world. We are called to accompany, console, and encourage the suffering and marginalized where they are—which is why we must go down deeply and thickly into the particulars of people and their lives. Platitudes or outrage seems almost inevitable if you are not familiar with the particulars of a person's life.

At present something is not right. We are striving to articulate truth without recourse to love. This is an intolerable situation. Are we more worried about orthodoxy or being in proximity and sharing the hope of the new life in Messiah? This kind of renewal comes at the edge of our structures. How do we do this right, so we do not damage our ability to minister to and impact real followers of God who are gay and who love Him?

We have a missional opportunity and thus I must extend myself to people who want to be accountable and in covenant. We will hear differently from Scripture. But we should agree that God's profound yearning in Jesus is "to seek and to save that which was lost." I believe this is an opportune moment for the church to boldly proclaim a pastoral, grace-filled readiness to include both homosexuals and heterosexuals within the blessing of a marriage covenant designed to be healthy and God-honoring.

For my own part, I have a firm commitment to the authority of the Scriptures. I strive to be faithfully obedient to Jesus. I also know that I must daringly venture out into this new territory. I must embrace the missional opportunity to those who are different and who desire to live in account-able, covenanted ways. I want to be generous and open while holding on to certain religious convictions, to treat people as I would wish to be treated.

I desire to engage and interact in such a way that people will know that God himself is our peace. I cannot give up our convictions about the gospel nor do I apologize for that kind of exclusion. My conviction remains that marriage and sexuality are sacred. I wish to be respected in this commitment and acknowledge the mystery of human sexuality. Yet I also do not expect that people must change their sexual orientation to follow Jesus. Orientation within the limits of covenant is morally neutral, and grace has no space for boundaries.

The power of God's love is superior to the defeating power of judgment. Where we draw that line may be in dispute—but may it not be disputed that we seek to honor and obey the great commandment and in doing for others that we would do for ourselves.

Clearly, there exists the possibility of genuine, reasoned, substantive debate over the rightness of same-sex marriage. I do not feel it is proper to take cheap shots against Christian tradition. I equally believe that I have earned the right to have an opinion by working through my tradition and trying to understand it, however poorly, at its deepest level. I ask to be treated respectfully and mercifully in communities where my worldview is not shared, as I would do to others.

Gay people are not going anywhere, and we absolutely cannot ask people who are different to violate their own particularity. Reducing people to their sexuality infringes on the complexity and richness of the human person. We must remember that difference is not a disease—it is difference. Can we communicate and engage with difference in loving ways that preserve human dignity? If homosexuality is inherent then barring that person from opportunities and human relationships prevents that person from thriving. This is a catastrophe, as is the fact that so many of us Christians have lost proximity with our gay family and friends.

In place of such an intense focus on sexual orientation, I invite all people to reflect on our spiritual orientation, toward God and toward our fellow human beings. When we do this, we also submit ourselves, replete with flaws and beauty, to God and his way of living as revealed in the teachings of Jesus.

Workbook Questions

1. In the opening story of this chapter, the pastor made what some would see as a radical choice. What do you think the pastor ought to have done, and why?

2. What do you think of the connection made between "disability and difference" and "difference in sexuality"? Would you make the same connection the author does? Why or why not?

3. Must orthodoxy mean that we cannot be proximate to sexual difference?

12

Conclusion

Rethinking Difference

As Rafi entered elementary and middle school, he was subjected to all means of tests: IQ tests, psychological tests, developmental tests, and reading tests. The results of these tests were sent to the department of education. The school board used these results to assign resources for Rafi, and we used these results to get benefits for him.

There is neither ability nor reason to deny the reality of human difference. But society is eager to measure, categorize, organize, and label difference, and with these, to control it and endow difference with meaning. Undoubtedly this control has provided a better life for Rafi and for many with disabilities, but at the same time I find myself a bit uneasy about the "classification and pigeon-holing of people for the efficacy of our health, education, immigration and employment systems."[1]

Measurement is not disinterested. Measurement is a process of categorization and looking for meaning. Measurement is ideological because it introduces value into the range of human differences, by placing them in some kind of order. I wondered about how Rafi was measured and if how he was measured can influence the meanings that follow from this process of measurement.

David Hiles says that

> as soon as we focus on the theorizing of human differences in this way, i.e., on the meaning of human differences, we must confront a

1. Hiles, "Human Diversity," 1.

> fundamental problem. The problem is that the meanings of human
> differences are not inherently fixed but are open to manipulation.
> Where they do become apparently fixed, then this is largely the
> consequence of ideological processes at work. But this problem
> is precisely the issue. It is a serious blind spot for psychology . . .[2]

The meaning of Rafi's difference often becomes focused on the categories of the measurement and study of his intelligence, personality, achievement, ability, and disability. This might be useful for society, but it seems
inattentive to his reality.

Existential thinkers like Heidegger and Levinas recognize that we live
in a world of "others" and that we must learn to recognize their inherent
humanity. Victor Shepherd says this is essential for making sense of Heidegger's understanding of the person: "To apprehend him at all is always
to apprehend him as human."[3] The meaning of Rafi's difference must be
something more than how the government assigns resources.

Human difference is in my face. Even though I benefit from it, I am
not interested in our classification systems for people for the sake of our
systems. My own interest is in Rafi's humanity and his enablement. Rafi
is here with the rest of us. To be human is to be here with everybody else.

Does Rafi know this? I do not think so. When he is in bed getting
ready to sleep and when I wake him in the morning, I often wonder what
he's thinking. About the meaning of his life? His hopes and dreams? What
I am certain of is that he knows that he is cared for and loved, and he loves
others. That must be enough. Beyond that, I know that he cares about his
family and his routines, and this gives him hope and meaning, and calms
his own anxiety.

I am not sure where that anxiety comes from. I ask him about it often
when he seems to be in a dark place: "Is something bothering you?" "What's
wrong?" "Are you anxious?" Without exception he says, "I don't know." I
think this is true. He does not know how to analyze these emotions, and he
reacts to them physically—he shuts down, holds his ears, crosses his arms,
or sometimes moans. It must be hard not being able to express yourself
when you are feeling something that you do not understand. He cannot
regulate it. I feel sad for him that he cannot express his needs and receive
comfort. Sometimes a hug seems to help.

2. Hiles, "Human Diversity," 2.
3. Shepherd, *Committed Self,* 274.

I have come to terms with the demands of living responsibly with Rafi for as long as I can. He has needs that are sometimes disturbing and will never end. It is not his power that leads me, that makes me responsible, but his vulnerability and his need, and the fear I have of his suffering. Rafi cannot conceptualize this, and no matter how responsible I already have been, I cannot be responsible enough. Rafi is the ongoing source of my ethics and sense of responsibility.[4] Living with Rafi challenges me every day with three fundamental questions:

1. What is it that I have decided that I would never do?
2. What is it that I have decided that I must do?
3. What kind of person do I want to be?

Concluding Thoughts on Rethinking Difference

As I reflect on my experience with difference, I think about the attitudes towards difference that I have encountered among people. Calling someone "different" often names a mode of oppression or injustice. The boundaries of the term "disabled" are endless and it is hard to get close to the word.

What really matters is not whether or how human differences can be measured, but the way in which these differences take on meanings. "Disabled" is a negativized term of difference positioned in relation to a norm. I challenge you to think about what or who represents normality. We have certain ideas about normalcy which we consent to, but at the basic level there is no norm, there are just differences and predispositions. The norm is difference. We choose certain criteria, and judge some forms of difference to be acceptable, while others are not. Assumptions are made about what it means to be human. I am eager to question our conceptions of "normal" and break down the binary distinction we make between "normal" and "different."

Our common human experience of embodied difference only underscores the importance of approaching the biblical texts through this lens. What would it look like to read the sacred text through a lens of human difference and how would this underscore enrich our understanding of humanity and human limits?

---

4. Edelglass, Hatley, and Diehm, "Introduction." Levinas' notion of the Other and my responsibility has helped me think through my obligation.

Proximity and starting from the particular can help to free us from fear and ensure that our ethics are grounded in the real lives, hopes, and challenges of other embodied humans, created in the image of God.

When you are thinking about Rafi, start with Rafi.

138

Workbook Questions

1. The author explains that living with Rafi forces him to ask essential questions about who he is and what he must do. What in your life forces you to ask fundamental questions of yourself on a regular basis?

2. How would you describe the relationship between disability and difference?

Bibliography

Block, Jennie Weiss. *Copious Hosting: A Theology of Access for People with Disabilities.* New York: Continuum, 2002.

Bonhoeffer, Dietrich. *The Cost of Discipleship.* 1937. Reprint, London: SCM, 2015.

———. *Creation and Fall; Temptation: Two Biblical Studies.* 1933. Reprint, New York: Simon & Schuster, 1997.

———. *Life Together: A Discussion of Christian Fellowship.* 1939. Reprint, San Francisco: Harper, 1978.

Brueggemann, Walter. *Spirituality of the Psalms.* Minneapolis: Fortress, 2001.

Canada Public Health Services. "Key Statistics." https://www.canada.ca/en/public-health/services/publications/healthy-living/suicide-canada-key-statistics-infographic.html.

———. "Suicide Prevention." https://www.canada.ca/en/public-health/services/publications/healthy-living/suicide-prevention-framework.html.

Canadian Down Syndrome Society. https://cdss.ca.

Carpenter, Humphrey, and Christopher Tolkien, eds. *The Letters of J. R. R. Tolkien.* 1981. Reprint, London: Harper Collins, 2006.

Chambers, Oswald. "God's Silence—Then What? | My Utmost for His Highest." Utmost.org, 2015. https://utmost.org/god%E2%80%99s-silence%E2%80%94-then-what/.

Chicago Tribune. "Why 'Million Dollar Baby' infuriates the disabled." February 2, 2005. https://www.chicagotribune.com/news/ct-xpm-2005-2-02-502020017-story.html.

Couser, Thomas G. "Disability as Diversity: A Difference with a Difference." *Ilha Do Desterro: A Journal of English Language, Literatures in English and Cultural Studies,* no. 48 (2005) 95–113. Redalyc, https://www.redalyc.org/articulo.oa?id=478348686004.

Craigie, Peter C. *The Book of Deuteronomy.* Grand Rapids: Eerdmans, 1976.

Creamer, Deborah Beth. *Disability and Christian Theology: Embodied Limits and Constructive Possibilities.* New York: Oxford University Press, 2009.

Davis, John Jefferson. *Evangelical Ethics.* Phillipsburg, NJ: Presbyterian and Reformed, 1985.

Du Bois, W. E. B. "Strivings of the Negro People." *The Atlantic,* August 1897. https://www.theatlantic.com/magazine/archive/1897/08/strivings-of-the-negro-people/305446/.

Edelglass, William, James Hatley, and Christian Diehm. "Introduction: Facing Nature after Levinas." In *Additional Information Facing Nature: Levinas and Environmental*

Thought, edited by William Edelglass, James Hatley, and Christian Diehm, 1–10. Pittsburgh: Duquesne University Press, 2012.

Edersheim, Alfred. *The Life and Times of Jesus the Messiah*. McLean, VA: MacDonald, 1883.

Eiesland, Nancy L. *The Disabled God: Toward a Liberatory Theology of Disability*. Nashville: Abingdon, 1994.

Estes, Joel D. "Imperfection in Paradise: Reading Genesis 2 through the Lens of Disability and a Theology of Limits." *Horizons in Biblical Theology* 38, no. 1 (April 19, 2016) 1–21. https://doi.org/10.1163/18712207–12341313.

Founders Archives. https://founders.archives.gov/documents/Washington/05-06-02-0135.

Genovese, Eugene D. *Roll, Jordan, Roll: The World the Slaves Made*. New York: Vintage, 1976.

Gladwell, Malcolm. "John Rock's Error." *The New Yorker*, March 5, 2000. https://www.newyorker.com/magazine/2000/03/13/john-rocks-error.

Gustafson, James M. *Theology and Christian Ethics*. Philadelphia: Pilgrim, 1974.

Hauerwas, Stanley. "Community and Diversity: The Tyranny of Normality." *Journal of Religion, Disability & Health* 8, no. 3–4 (February 24, 2005) 37–43. https://doi.org/10.1300/j095v08n03_05.

———. *The Hauerwas Reader*. Edited by John Berkman and Michael G. Cartwright. London: Duke University Press, 2005.

———. *Matthew*. Grand Rapids: Brazos, 2006.

Health Canada. "Annual Report." https://www.canda.ca/en/health-canada/services/publications/health-system-services/annual-report-medical-assistance-dying-2022.html.

Heschel, Abraham Joshua. *God in Search of Man: A Philosophy of Judaism*. New York: Farrar, Straus and Cudahy, 1955.

———. *The Sabbath: Its Meaning for Modern Man*. New York: Farrar, Straus and Giroux, 1951.

Hiles, David. "Human Diversity, and the Meaning of Difference." Presented at the Tenth European Congress of Psychology. Prague, CZ, 2007.

Hull, John. *Touching the Rock: An Experience of Blindness*. London: SPCK, 2016.

Jesuits of Canada. "The Jesuits & Jean Vanier, the 'Giant of God's Kindness.'" May 9, 2019. https://jesuits.ca/stories/the-jesuits-jean-vanier-the-giant-of-gods-kindness/.

Keener, Craig S. "The Cause of Blindness (9:2–5)." In *The Gospel of John*. Vol. 1. Kindle ed. Grand Rapids: Baker Academic, 2003.

Kohl, Marvin. "Beneficent Euthanasia." *Humanist* 34, no. 4 (1974) 9–11.

Levenson, Jon D. *Creation and the Persistence of Evil: The Jewish Drama of Divine Omnipotence*. Princeton: Princeton University Press, 1994.

Lewis, C. S. *God in the Dock*. London: Collins, 1971.

———. *A Grief Observed*. New York: Bantam, 1961.

———. *Mere Christianity*. New York: Macmillan, 1952.

———. *The Screwtape Letters*. New York: Macmillan, 1943.

———. *The Voyage of the Dawn Treader*. New York: Macmillan, 1952.

———. "The Weight of Glory." In *The Weight of Glory and Other Essays*, 1–15. New York: Macmillan, 1949.

London, Daniel. "Judging God: Learning from the Jewish Tradition of Protest against God." *Journal of Comparative Theology* 6, no. 1 (June 2016) 15–31.

Mansfield, C., et al. "Termination Rates after Prenatal Diagnosis of Down Syndrome, Spinal Bifida, Anencephaly, and Turner and Klinefelter Syndromes: A Systematic Literature Review." *Prenatal Diagnosis* 19 (1999) 808–12.

Marucchi, Orazio. "Archaeology of the Cross and Crucifix." In *The Catholic Encyclopedia,* vol. 4. New York: Robert Appleton, 1908. www.newadvent.ord/cathen/04517a.htm.

McCrum, Robert. "My Old and New Lives." *The New Yorker Magazine,* May 27, 1996, 112–18.

Moltmann, Jürgen. "Liberate Yourselves by Accepting One Another." In *Human Disability and the Service of God: Reassessing Religious Practice,* edited by Nancy L. Eiesland and Don E. Saliers, 105–22. Nashville: Abingdon, 1998.

Murray, John. *The Epistle to the Romans.* 1959. Reprint, Grand Rapids: Eerdmans, 1997.

Prager, Dennis. "Cahill's Gift." *First Things,* November 1998. https://www.firstthings.com/article/1998/11/cahills-gift.

Press Association. "Richard Dawkins Apologises for Causing Storm with Down's Syndrome Tweet." *The Guardian,* August 21, 2014. https://www.theguardian.com/science/2014/aug/21/richard-dawkins-apologises-downs-syndrome-tweet.

Presson, A. F., et al. "Current Estimate of Down Syndrome Population Prevalence in the United States." *Journal of Pediatrics* 163, no. 4 (2013) 1163–68.

Radner, Ephraim. "Divine Irreplaceability." Covenant, December 15, 2020. https://livingchurch.org/covenant/2020/12/15/divine-irreplaceability/

———. *Leviticus.* Grand Rapids: Brazos, 2008.

———. "The Psychedelic Body: Finding God in the Flesh." February 27, 2019. https://www.youtube.com/watch?v=RZL-qTOha1I.

———. *Time and the Word: Figural Reading of the Christian Scriptures.* Grand Rapids: Eerdmans, 2016.

———. *A Time to Keep: Theology, Mortality, and the Shape of a Human Life.* Waco, TX: Baylor University Press, 2016.

Rao, Tejal. "What Is Hospitality? The Current Answer Doesn't Work." *New York Times,* April 13, 2021. https://www.nytimes.com/2021/04/13/dining/restaurant-hospitality.html.

Reynolds, Thomas E. *Vulnerable Communion: A Theology of Disability and Hospitality.* Grand Rapids: Brazos, 2008.

Rigney, Joe. "C. S. Lewis and the Role of the Physical Body in Prayer." Crossway, April 23, 2018. https://www.crossway.org/articles/cs-lewis-and-the-role-of-the-physical-body-in-prayer.

Robinson, Rich. *Christ in the Sabbath.* Chicago: Moody, 2014.

Sacks, Jonathan. *The Dignity of Difference: How to Avoid the Clash of Civilizations.* London: Continuum, 2007.

Santos, Narry. "Biblical Bases of Hospitality." In *Beyond Hospitality: Migration, Multiculturalism, and the Church,* edited by Charles A. Cook, Lauren Goldbeck, and Lorajoy Tira-Dimangondayao, 39–47. Toronto: Tyndale Academic, 2020.

Schmutzer, Andrew, and Alice Mathews. "Genesis 1–11 and Work." Theology of Work Project, June 11, 2013. https://www.theologyofwork.org/old-testament/genesis-1-11-and-work#limits-genesis-23-217.

Serving People with Disabilities (SPD). "Disability in Fashion," April 2, 2015. https://spd.org.sg/disability-in-fashion/.

Shepherd, Victor A. *The Committed Self: An Introduction to Existentialism for Christians.* Toronto: BPS, 2015.

———. "'My Ministry Is Dearer to Me than Life'—Sermons & Writings of Victor Shepherd." victorshepherd.ca, June 2008. https://victorshepherd.ca/my-ministry-is-dearer-to-me-than-life/.

Shweik, Susan. "The Voice of 'Reason." In *Beauty Is a Verb: The New Poetry of Disability*, edited by Jennifer Bartlett, Sheila Black, and Michael Northern, 67–80. El Paso: Cinco Puntos, 2011.

Singer, Peter. *Practical Ethics*. New York: Cambridge University Press, 1969.

Stiff, Anthony J. "The Abiding Value of John Calvin's Eucharistic Theology for Disability Theology." *Calvin Theological Journal* 54, no. 1 (2019) 129–45.

Stiker, Henri-Jacques. *A History of Disability*. New ed. Ann Arbor: University of Michigan Press, 2019.

Swinton, John. "Breaking the Mold with John Swinton." Podcast. Sanctuary Mental Health Ministries, January 30, 2020. https://sanctuarymentalhealth.org/2020/01/30/john-swinton/.

———. Disability, Time, and the Spiritual Dimension of Health." Interview by Tripp Fuller, January 17, 2018. https://trippfuller.com/2018/01/17/disability-time-and-the-spiritual-dimension-of-health-with-john-swinton/.

———. "J. J. Thiessen Lectures—Lecture 2." October 14, 2014. https://www.youtube.com/watch?v=TJo5kodHPes.

———. "Many Bodies, Many Worlds." *Disability*. Christian Reflection: A Series in Faith and Ethics. Center for Christian Ethics at Baylor University (2012) 18–24.

———. "Who Is the God We Worship? Theologies of Disability; Challenges and New Possibilities." *International Journal of Practical Theology* 14, no. 2 (January 2011) 273–307. https://doi.org/10.1515/ijpt.2011.020.

Tataryn, Myroslaw, and Maria Truchan-Tataryn. *Discovering Trinity in Disability: A Theology for Embracing Difference*. Maryknoll, NY: Orbis, 2013.

Vanier, Jean. *Becoming Human*. Toronto: House of Anansi, 1998.

Wannenwetsch, Bernd. "'My Strength Is Made Perfect in Weakness': Bonhoeffer and the War over Disabled Life." In *Disability in the Christian Tradition*, edited by Brian Brock and John Swinton, 353–90. Grand Rapids: Eerdmans, 2012.

Watson, Timothy. "Is Heschel's Sabbath Biblical?" *Andrews University Seminary Studies* 40, no. 2 (2022) 265–72.

White, William. *Notes and Queries*. Vol. 8. Oxford: Oxford University Press, 1853.

Wingren, Gustaf, and Carl C. Rasmussen. *Luther on Vocation*. Eugene, OR: Wipf & Stock, 2004.